FOLLICULAR LYMPHOMA

A survival guide for patients

Dr. Bhratri Bhushan,
MD, DM

Copyright © 2026 Dr. Bhratri Bhushan

Copyright © 2026 by Dr. Bhratri Bhushan

All rights reserved. No part of this publication may be reproduced, distributed, or transmitted in any form or by any means, including photocopying, recording, or other electronic or mechanical methods, without the prior written permission of the publisher, except in the case of brief quotations embodied in critical reviews and certain other noncommercial uses permitted by copyright law.

For permission requests, write to the publisher, addressed Attention: Permissions Coordinator, at the address:

A30, Ananta institute of medical sciences,
Rajsamand, Rajasthan, India 313202
Email: www.bhratri@gmail.com

This work is provided as is, and the author and the publisher disclaim any and all warranties, express or implied, including any warranties as to accuracy, comprehensiveness, or currency of the content of this work.

To the maximum extent permitted under applicable law, no responsibility is assumed by the publisher for any injury and/or damage to persons or property as a matter of products liability, negligence law or otherwise, or from any reference to or use by any person of this work.

CONTENTS

Title Page
Copyright
Preface
Chapter 1: The Basics of the Lymphatic System   1
Chapter 2: What is Follicular Lymphoma?   4
Chapter 3: Decoding Your Pathology Report   7
Chapter 4: The Staging and Grading Puzzle   10
Chapter 5: The FL Ecosystem: Mutations and Microenvironments   21
Chapter 6: The "Watch and Wait" Strategy (Active Surveillance)   24
Chapter 7: Treatment Options (The "Menu" of Care)   32
Chapter 8: Relapse and Transformation   36
Chapter 9: Emerging Frontiers: CAR-T and Bispecifics   39
Chapter 10: An Algorithmic Approach to Treating Follicular Lymphoma   42
Chapter 11: The Lymphoma-Friendly Kitchen   60
Chapter 12: Movement as Medicine   63
Chapter 13: The Art of Restorative Sleep   66

Chapter 14: Neutropenic Living: Staying Safe in a Germ-Filled World — 69

Chapter 15: Integrative Therapies: Beyond the Prescription — 73

Chapter 16: Cracking the Code of Cancer Fatigue — 76

Chapter 17: Managing the "Queasies": Nausea & Digestive Health — 79

Chapter 18: The Fog: Coping with "Chemo Brain" — 82

Chapter 19: Taming the Fire: Neuropathy & Nerve Pain — 85

Chapter 20: Skin, Hair, and Nails: The External Journey — 88

Chapter 21: Mouth Sores and Taste Changes — 91

Chapter 22: The "Watch and Wait" Paradox — 94

Chapter 23: Scanxiety: Navigating the Two-Week Wait — 97

Chapter 24: Difficult Conversations: Talking to Family and Children — 100

Chapter 25: Intimacy and Sexuality During Treatment — 103

Chapter 26: The Organized Patient: Managing Records and Results — 107

Chapter 27: Career and Cancer: To Work or Not to Work? — 110

Chapter 28: The Lymphoma Traveler's Guide — 113

Chapter 29: Financial Toxicity: Navigating Insurance and Assistance	116
Chapter 30: The Caregiver's Compass	120
About The Author	123

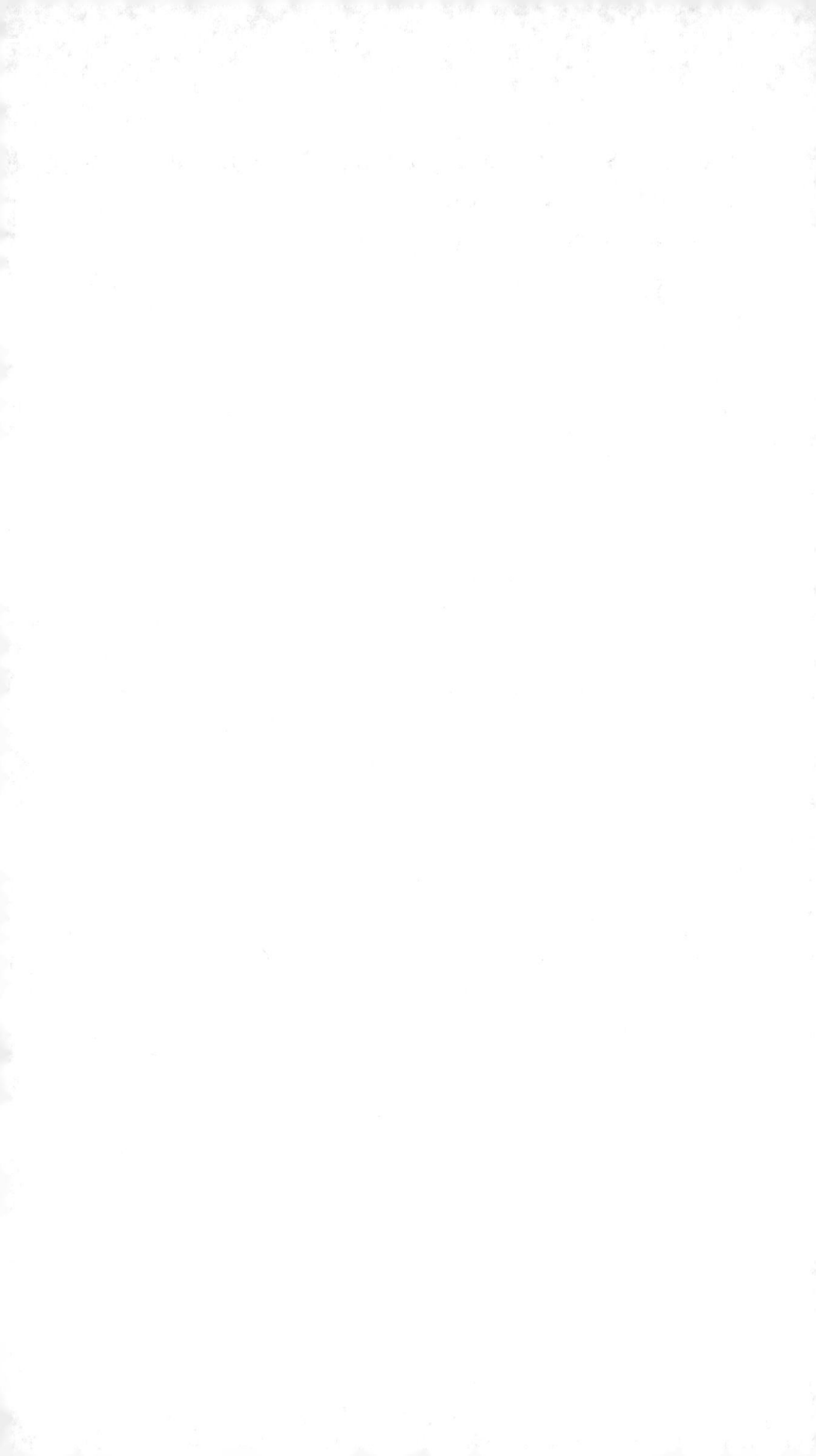

PREFACE

Writing a book about Follicular Lymphoma (FL) is a bit like trying to map a landscape that is constantly shifting. As an oncologist, I spend my days looking at PET scans and pathology reports, but those are just the "data points" of a life. They don't capture the heavy silence in the room when I tell someone they have a cancer that we might not even treat yet. They don't capture the exhaustion of a parent trying to play with their children while their mind is stuck on a Ki-67 percentage.

I've sat across from hundreds of people at this exact crossroads. Usually, there is a specific look in a patient's eyes—a mix of "Why me?" and "What now?" Medical textbooks are excellent at answering the first question with biology, but they are notoriously bad at the second. They can tell you the dosage of Rituximab, but they won't tell you how to handle the "metallic mouth" that makes your favorite meal taste like a handful of coins, or how to explain to your family that you aren't "lazy"—you're experiencing a type of fatigue that sleep cannot fix.

This is the book I wish I could hand every patient

the moment we finish our first consultation.

Follicular Lymphoma is a unique beast. It is often labeled "indolent" or "slow-growing," which sounds almost gentle, doesn't it? But there is nothing gentle about the psychological "slow burn" of living with a chronic malignancy. It is a marathon, not a sprint. It requires a different kind of stamina—not just physical, but emotional and philosophical.

In these pages, I am going to do two things for you:

1. **I will be your clinician.** I've laid out the hard science—the treatments, the guidelines, and the new frontiers like CAR-T and bispecific antibodies—because knowledge is the only real antidote to the "darkness" of a new diagnosis.

2. **I will be your guide.** We are going to step out of the clinic and into your kitchen, your bedroom, and your workplace. We'll talk about how to eat when nothing sounds good, how to move your body when you're tired, and how to navigate the "Watch and Wait" period without losing your mind.

We live in an era of medicine where we are getting very good at keeping people alive. Now, we need to focus on making sure that life is actually worth living. You are more than a collection of B-cells; you are a person with a story that is still being written.

CHAPTER 1: THE BASICS OF THE LYMPHATIC SYSTEM

To understand what a B-cell is, we first have to look at the lymphatic system not as a series of static tubes, but as the body's secondary highway —a vital, circulating network that works quietly in the shadow of the blood vessels. While your heart pumps blood with a rhythmic, forceful beat, the lymphatic system is much more subtle. It's a drainage and surveillance network that collects excess fluid from your tissues and filters it through small, bean-shaped hubs we call lymph nodes. It is within these nodes that the real "magic" of the immune system happens, and it's where our protagonist, the B-cell, waits for its moment to shine.

Think of the immune system as a highly specialized security force. Most of the cells you hear about, like neutrophils or macrophages, are the "first responders." They are tough, general-purpose cells that rush to the site of an injury or infection and start cleaning up whatever doesn't belong. They are effective, but they aren't particularly surgical. This is where the B-cell comes in. A B-cell is a type of white blood cell, specifically a lymphocyte, that represents the "intelligence" wing of your immunity. If the first responders are the patrol officers, the B-cells are the specialists who create the blueprints for specific "keys"—better known as antibodies—designed to lock onto and neutralize a very specific enemy.

Every B-cell is born in the bone marrow, which is essentially the body's primary training academy for blood cells. While they are still "naive," meaning they haven't yet met a germ they need to fight, they circulate through the lymph and blood, decorated with unique receptors on their surface. Each B-cell is essentially programmed to recognize one, and only one, specific shape. There might be a B-cell in your body right now that is perfectly shaped to recognize a specific protein on a flu virus, and another meant for a common bacterium. They wait in the lymph nodes, like sentries at a gate, for their specific "target" to float by in the lymphatic fluid.

When a B-cell finally encounters the specific invader it was designed for, it undergoes a dramatic transformation. It doesn't just attack; it clones itself rapidly, turning into a massive factory known as a plasma cell. These plasma cells are the heavy hitters of the immune world. Their sole job is to pump out thousands of antibodies per second into the bloodstream. These antibodies are like precision-guided stickers. They fly through the body and latch onto the virus or bacteria, doing two things: they physically block the germ from entering your healthy cells, and they act as a "glow-in-the-dark" beacon that tells the rest of the immune system,

"This thing is dangerous—come destroy it."

This process is what we call the "adaptive" immune response. It's "adaptive" because it learns. Once the battle is over, most of those B-cells die off, but a few remain behind as "memory B-cells." These cells live for years, sometimes a lifetime. They remember exactly what that specific enemy looked like. This is why, if you encounter the same germ a second time, your body doesn't have to wait days to figure out a plan; the memory B-cells recognize it instantly and trigger a massive antibody response before you even feel a single symptom. This "memory" is the fundamental principle behind how vaccines work—they give your B-cells a "preview" of the enemy so they can build their defense system without you ever having to get sick.

In a perfectly functioning system, this is a beautiful, self-regulating cycle. The lymphatic system gathers the evidence, the B-cells identify the threat, the antibodies neutralize it, and the memory cells keep a record for the future. It is a constant, invisible conversation between your cells and the environment, a testament to the body's incredible ability to not just survive, but to remember and grow stronger with every challenge it faces.

CHAPTER 2: WHAT IS FOLLICULAR LYMPHOMA?

To truly understand follicular lymphoma, it helps to first step away from the frightening weight of the word "cancer" and look at how the disease actually behaves in the body. If you think back to how B-cells are supposed to work—as disciplined sentries waiting in the lymph nodes—follicular lymphoma represents a shift in that discipline. In this condition, certain B-cells begin to multiply in a way that is slow, quiet, and persistent. They don't rush through the body like an aggressive infection; instead, they cluster together in small, circular patterns called "follicles" within the lymph nodes. This characteristic growth pattern is exactly where the name "follicular" comes from.

When doctors talk about this disease, they often use words like "indolent" or "chronic." In plain English, "indolent" essentially means lazy or slow-moving. Unlike aggressive lymphomas that demand immediate, intensive intervention, follicular lymphoma often takes its time. It is a marathon, not a sprint. This is why many patients are surprised to learn that their treatment plan might involve "watchful waiting" or active surveillance. It's a counterintuitive idea—knowing a cancer is present but choosing not to attack it with everything at once—but it's based on the reality that this is a chronic condition. Much like high blood pressure or diabetes, the goal isn't always a one-time "cure" in the traditional sense, but rather managing the disease over many years, or even decades, so that it doesn't interfere with a long and full life.

However, not all follicular lymphomas are identical, which brings us to the concept of "grading." When a pathologist looks at a sample of these cells under a microscope, they are essentially counting how many large, fast-growing cells (called centroblasts) are mixed in with the smaller, slower-moving ones. This isn't about how much cancer is in the body —that's "staging"—but rather about the "flavor" or personality of the cells themselves. We generally categorize them into three grades: 1, 2, and 3a.

Grades 1 and 2 are often grouped together because they look and act very similarly. They are composed mostly of those smaller, sleepy cells. If your diagnosis is Grade 1 or 2, it confirms that the disease is behaving in that typical, slow-moving, indolent fashion. Grade 3a is a bit more of a middle ground; it shows a higher number of those larger cells, suggesting the disease might be slightly more active, though it is still generally managed under the follicular lymphoma umbrella. There is also a Grade 3b, but that is often treated more like an aggressive lymphoma, as it has crossed a threshold where the cells are moving much faster.

It is important to remember that having a "chronic" disease is a double-edged sword. On one hand, it means the urgency is often lower, giving you and your medical team time to make thoughtful, unhurried decisions. On the other hand, because the cells are slow-moving, they aren't always as vulnerable to traditional chemotherapy, which specifically targets fast-dividing cells. This is why the focus in follicular lymphoma has shifted so heavily toward smarter, targeted therapies that can keep the B-cells in check over the long haul. Understanding that this is a slow-motion process is the first step in stripping away the panic and replacing it with a clear-eyed strategy for the future.

CHAPTER 3: DECODING YOUR PATHOLOGY REPORT

When you receive a pathology report, it can feel like you've been handed a document written in a foreign language. It is dense, filled with alphanumeric codes and cryptic descriptions of cell shapes. But if we pull back the curtain, this report is actually a very detailed character profile of the lymphoma. It tells us not just what the disease is, but how it behaves and what tools we have to fight it. The first thing you'll usually see is a description of the "follicular" pattern itself. Under a microscope, instead of the lymph node looking like a chaotic, disorganized crowd, the B-cells are gathered into neat, circular islands. These are the "follicles." In a healthy node, these circles are where immune cells go to mature; in follicular lymphoma, the B-cells have essentially set up permanent camp there, refusing to leave and continuing to grow in these tight, recognizable clusters. This architectural layout is the signature that allows a pathologist to name the disease.

Once the physical structure is identified, the pathologist starts looking for "markers"—essentially molecular name tags on the surface of the cells. The most famous of these is **CD20**. Think of CD20 as a specific docking port that is found almost exclusively on B-cells. Seeing "CD20 positive" on your report is actually very good news. It confirms that the lymphoma is made of B-cells, and more importantly, it means the disease is "visible" to one of our most effective treatments: rituximab. Rituximab is a monoclonal antibody designed like a homing missile to find that CD20 dock, latch onto it, and signal the immune system to destroy the cell. Without that marker, our most targeted tool wouldn't know where to land.

Beyond the surface markers, the report will often mention **Ki-67**. This is a "proliferation index," which is a fancy way of saying it measures how many cells are currently in the process of dividing. If you think of the lymphoma as a car, Ki-67 tells us how much pressure is on the gas pedal. In most cases of follicular lymphoma, the Ki-67 percentage is quite low—perhaps 10% or 20%—which confirms the "indolent" or slow-moving nature we've discussed. If the number is higher, it suggests the cells are dividing more rapidly, which might influence how aggressively your doctor wants to approach treatment. It's a snapshot of the disease's current energy level.

You might also see a list of other markers like CD10 or BCL2. These are essentially "proof of identity" markers. For instance, BCL2 is a protein that normally tells a cell when it is time to die. In follicular lymphoma, a genetic "glitch" keeps this BCL2 switch stuck in the "on" position, effectively giving the B-cells an "immortality" signal. This is why the cells build up over time—not necessarily because they are growing at a lightning-fast pace, but because they have forgotten how to die when they are supposed to.

Reading these results can be overwhelming, but try to view the report as a roadmap rather than a verdict. Every positive marker and every percentage point provides a piece of the puzzle that helps your medical team tailor a plan specifically for you. It moves the conversation from "what is this?" to "how do we manage this specifically?" Having this level of detail is exactly what allows modern medicine to treat follicular lymphoma with such precision, ensuring that the treatment fits the disease's unique personality.

CHAPTER 4: THE STAGING AND GRADING PUZZLE

If the pathology report we discussed earlier is the "personality profile" of the disease, then staging is the "road map." In the world of follicular lymphoma, we use a framework called the Ann Arbor staging system. It's a bit of a classic, named after the city in Michigan where it was first standardized, and it essentially tracks how far the lymphoma has traveled along the body's lymphatic highway. To understand this map, you first have to visualize the diaphragm—that thin sheet of muscle that separates your chest from your abdomen. In staging, the diaphragm acts as the primary border control.

Stage I is when the lymphoma is found in just one spot—perhaps a single group of lymph nodes in the neck or the armpit. Stage II means it has moved to a second location, but importantly, both spots are still on the same side of the diaphragm (both above it in the chest/neck, or both below it in the abdomen). Once the disease is found on both sides of the diaphragm, we call it Stage III. Finally, Stage IV occurs when the lymphoma has moved outside the lymphatic system entirely, settling in places like the liver, the lungs, or most commonly, the bone marrow.

Now, this is where things get interesting—and where many people feel a justifiable sense of panic that needs to be addressed. In the world of solid tumors, like lung or breast cancer, "Stage IV" is a heavy, frightening term that usually implies the cancer has become "metastatic" and is much more difficult to treat. But follicular lymphoma is a different beast entirely. Because B-cells are naturally designed to circulate through your entire body as part of your immune surveillance, it is incredibly common—in fact, it's the norm—for follicular lymphoma to be Stage IV at the very moment it is diagnosed. About 80% of patients start at Stage III or IV.

In this context, Stage IV doesn't mean the disease is "terminal" in the way people often fear. It simply reflects the nature of the lymphatic system itself. Think of it like a dandelion in a field; if you see the seeds floating in several different corners, it doesn't necessarily mean the field is ruined— it just means the process is systemic. In follicular lymphoma, someone with Stage IV disease can often live for decades with the right management. The stage tells the doctor *where* the disease is, but it doesn't necessarily tell them how "mean" the disease is. That's why we look at the grade (the cell's personality) and the stage (the location) together to solve the puzzle.

You might also see letters like "A" or "B" attached to your stage. This is a simple way of noting whether you are experiencing what we call "systemic symptoms." "A" means you feel generally fine, while "B" indicates you've had significant fevers, drenching night sweats, or unexplained weight loss. These details, combined with the map of the disease, help us decide if we should simply keep a close eye on things or if it's time to intervene with treatment. Staging isn't a countdown; it's a tool for strategy, ensuring we aren't using a sledgehammer where a lighter touch—or no touch at all—is required.

*The "gold standard" roadmap
for the curious reader*

1. The Biopsy Strategy: No Shortcuts

The guidelines are very clear: to get a correct diagnosis, the doctor needs a "big picture" look at the lymph node.

- A. **The Gold Standard:** An **Excisional Biopsy** (removing the whole node) or an **Incisional Biopsy** (removing a large piece) is preferred. This is because the pathologist needs to see the "architecture"—how the cells are organized into those circular "follicles."

- B. **The "No-Go":** A Fine-Needle Aspiration (FNA) is officially **insufficient**. It's like trying to understand a complex jigsaw puzzle by looking at just two or three pieces; it doesn't give enough context.

C. **The Alternative:** If a node is hard to reach (like deep in the abdomen), a **Core Needle Biopsy** (a thicker needle that takes a "plug" of tissue) is acceptable, especially if they take multiple samples and combine them with other tests.

2. The "Naming" Revolution (WHO vs. ICC)

There are two different classification systems: the **WHO (World Health Organization)** and the **ICC (International Consensus Classification)**.

A. **Grades 1, 2, and 3A:** These are the classic, slow-moving versions. The WHO now simply calls these **"Classic Follicular Lymphoma (cFL)."**

B. **Grade 3B:** This is the "aggressive" cousin. Even though it has "follicular" in the name, it behaves more like **DLBCL** (Diffuse Large B-Cell Lymphoma) and is usually treated with a more intensive "hammer" (stronger chemotherapy).

C. **The "Rule of Aggression":** If a biopsy shows *any* area of DLBCL mixed in with the follicular cells, the whole thing is treated as the more aggressive disease. We don't ignore the faster-growing part.

3. The "Fingerprint" (Immunophenotyping)

To confirm it's actually Follicular Lymphoma, the lab looks for specific proteins (markers) on the surface of the cells.

- A. **The Signature:** A typical case is **CD20+**, **CD10+**, and **BCL2+**.
- B. **BCL2 and t(14;18):** These are the "immortality" markers we've discussed before. If a patient is young and *lacks* these, the doctor has to look for rare variants, like "Pediatric-type" FL, which can actually occur in adults and often has a very good outlook.
- C. **Ki-67:** This is the "gas pedal" marker. If it's over **30%**, the disease might act a bit more aggressively, though the text notes that this doesn't necessarily mean you change the treatment plan right away.

4. Special Situations and Rare Variants

The text highlights a few versions that don't follow the classic rules:

- A. **dFL (Diffuse FL):** This version grows more in a "spread out" pattern rather than neat circles. It's often found in the groin (inguinal) area and has specific genetic mutations (like *STAT6*).
- B. **IRF4/MUM1 Rearrangement:** This is a very specific genetic "glitch." It often shows up in the "Waldeyer's Ring" (the tonsils and throat area), usually in younger people. It's locally aggressive but responds very well to treatment.

5. The "Body Scan": Physical Exam and Performance Status

The workup starts with the basics. The doctor checks "node-bearing areas"—the neck, armpits, and groin—but also looks at **Waldeyer's ring** (the tonsils and throat area), as lymphoma can hide there. They also check for an enlarged liver or spleen.

A. **Performance Status:** This is a simple score (often 0 to 5) that rates how well you can perform daily activities. It helps doctors decide if you can handle aggressive treatment or if a gentler approach is better. The ECOG Scale Breakdown:
   A. **Grade 0: Fully active.** You can carry on all pre-disease activities without restriction. If you were running 5Ks before your diagnosis and you still are, you are an ECOG 0.
   B. **Grade 1: Restricted in physically strenuous activity.** You are mobile and can perform light house or office work (e.g., light housework, office work). You might feel a bit more tired than usual, but you're still "up and about."
   C. **Grade 2: Up and about more than 50% of waking hours.** You are capable of all self-care but unable to carry out any work activities. This is the "pivot point" for many treatments; you

are ambulatory but spend a significant portion of the day resting.

D. **Grade 3: Capable of only limited self-care.** You are confined to a bed or chair more than 50% of your waking hours. This usually indicates that the disease or treatment is taking a heavy physical toll.

E. **Grade 4: Completely disabled.** You cannot carry on any self-care and are totally confined to a bed or chair.

F. **Grade 5: Death.**

B. **B Symptoms:** They will ask if you've had drenching night sweats, unexplained fevers, or lost more than 10% of your body weight. The presence of these "B symptoms" often suggests the disease is more active.

6. The "Liquid Data": Blood Tests

The blood work tells the story of how your organs are coping.

A. **CBC and Metabolic Panel:** These check your "counts" (white cells, red cells, platelets) and your kidney and liver function.

B. **LDH (Lactate Dehydrogenase):** This is a key marker. If it's high, it often means the lymphoma cells are turning over quickly. It's a vital piece of the "FLIPI" score used to predict how the disease will behave.

C. **Hepatitis B Testing:** This is a mandatory safety step. Some lymphoma treatments (like Rituximab) can "wake up" a dormant Hepatitis B virus, which could cause liver failure. If you've ever been exposed, you may need preventative medication during treatment.

7. The "Map": PET/CT Scans

The **PET/CT scan** is the preferred tool for staging. While a standard CT shows the *size* of the nodes, the PET scan shows how *active* they are by measuring how much sugar (glucose) the cells are consuming.

1. **Stage I-II:** The disease is limited to one side of the diaphragm (e.g., just the neck or just the groin).
2. **Stage III-IV:** The disease is on both sides of the diaphragm or involves organs like the bone marrow or liver.

8. The "Selected Cases": Deep Dives

Not every patient needs these, but they are crucial in certain scenarios:

A. **Bone Marrow Biopsy:** Usually done if the doctor thinks you are Stage I or II and they want to be 100% sure it hasn't reached the marrow before suggesting localized radiation. It's also done if your blood counts are inexplicably low.

B. **Heart Health (ECHO/MUGA):** If the plan involves a "heavy-hitter" chemotherapy (like an anthracycline), they must check your heart's pumping strength (ejection fraction) first to ensure it can handle the stress.

C. **Beta-2-Microglobulin:** This is another "prognostic" marker used to calculate the **FLIPI-2** score, helping to categorize your risk level.

D. **Fertility Preservation:** Since some treatments can affect the ability to have children, this must be discussed *before* any therapy starts. Options like sperm banking or egg freezing are the standard recommendations here.

The outcome of this "Workup" determines which page of the manual the doctor turns to next. If you are Stage I or II, you might be looking at **Involved-Site Radiation Therapy (ISRT)**. If you are Stage III or IV, the conversation shifts to either **Active Surveillance** ("Watch and Wait") or systemic therapies.

Staging

When doctors talk about the "stage" of your lymphoma, they are essentially drawing a map of where the cells have traveled. We use the diaphragm

—the thin muscle that separates your chest from your abdomen—as the primary border. This helps us categorize the disease into two main buckets: **Limited** and **Advanced**.

Limited Disease: Stages I and II

In these early stages, the lymphoma is still "localized," meaning it hasn't traveled very far from its starting point.

A. **Stage I:** The lymphoma is found in only one lymph node group (like just the left side of your neck) or in a single organ outside the lymph nodes.

B. **Stage II:** The lymphoma is in two or more node groups, but they are all on the **same side** of the diaphragm. For example, you might have involvement in your neck and your armpit, but nothing below your waist.

C. **Stage II Bulky:** This is Stage II disease where at least one of the masses is large (typically **7.5 cm** or greater). Because of the size, we often treat this more like an advanced stage to be safe.

Advanced Disease: Stages III and IV

Advanced stages mean the lymphoma has used the "highway" of the lymphatic system to cross into different territories of the body.

A. **Stage III:** The lymphoma is found in node groups on **both sides** of the diaphragm. This might mean nodes are involved in both the chest and the abdomen, or the neck and the groin. If the spleen is involved alongside nodes above the diaphragm, it is also considered Stage III.

B. **Stage IV:** This represents the most extensive spread. Here, the lymphoma has moved into organs that aren't part of the lymphatic system, such as the liver, lungs, or bone marrow.

A Note on the "E" Designation

You might see a small letter **"E"** next to your stage (e.g., Stage IIE). This simply stands for "extranodal." It means the lymphoma started in a lymph node but has spread into a nearby organ or tissue that is right next to it. It doesn't necessarily change your stage from II to IV, but it tells the doctor exactly where the "neighborhood" of the cancer ends.

CHAPTER 5: THE FL ECOSYSTEM: MUTATIONS AND MICROENVIRONMENTS

To understand why follicular lymphoma behaves the way it does, we have to look past the individual cancer cell and examine the entire "neighborhood" it lives in. In medicine, we call this the microenvironment, and in follicular lymphoma, it is arguably just as important as the cancer itself. You see, most cancers are like invasive weeds that try to kill off everything around them to take over the garden. Follicular lymphoma is different; it's more like a needy houseguest that moves in and then convinces the rest of the household to wait on it hand and foot.

The story starts with a specific genetic "glitch" that occurs in almost every case of this disease —a translocation between chromosomes 14 and 18. This isn't something you were born with or something you can pass on to your children; it's a random error that happened in a single B-cell at some point in your life. This error flips a switch on a protein called BCL2. In a healthy cell, BCL2 is a regulator that tells a cell when its time is up, but in these B-cells, the switch gets stuck in the "on" position. The result isn't a cell that grows at a terrifying speed, but rather a cell that simply refuses to die. It's the "immortality" signal that allows these cells to slowly accumulate in the lymph nodes over years.

But the B-cell doesn't survive on its own. It creates a complex ecosystem within the lymph node, surrounding itself with healthy supporting cells like T-cells and follicular dendritic cells. In a normal immune response, these supporting cells would recognize an invader and attack it. In follicular lymphoma, the cancer cells actually "re-educate" these healthy neighbors. They send out chemical signals that trick the T-cells into protecting the lymphoma instead of destroying it. It's a bit like a master manipulator who convinces the security guards to stand outside *their* door specifically. This is why the disease is so persistent; it isn't just a mass of bad cells, but a functioning, hijacked community that provides the cancer with growth signals and a shield against the body's natural defenses.

This "neighborhood" dynamic also explains why the disease is so unpredictable. Sometimes the ecosystem is stable, and the lymphoma stays "indolent" or sleepy for a decade. Other times, the cancer cells pick up additional mutations—new genetic typos—that allow them to become less dependent on their neighbors and more aggressive on their own. This constant dialogue between the mutations inside the cell and the environment outside the cell is the heartbeat of the disease. It's a delicate balance of power, and understanding this ecosystem is exactly how we're developing new treatments. Instead of just trying to kill the B-cell with "brute force" chemotherapy, we are now using drugs that "un-mask" the cancer, telling the surrounding T-cells to wake up and realize that the houseguest they've been protecting is actually an intruder.

CHAPTER 6: THE "WATCH AND WAIT" STRATEGY (ACTIVE SURVEILLANCE)

The concept of "Watch and Wait"—or as many doctors now prefer to call it, "Active Surveillance"—is perhaps the most difficult hurdle for a patient to clear emotionally. We are conditioned to believe that if you find a problem, you fix it immediately. If there is an intruder in the house, you don't sit in the living room and watch them; you call the police. So, when a doctor looks at a diagnosis of follicular lymphoma and suggests doing absolutely nothing in terms of active treatment, it can feel like a dereliction of duty. It sounds passive, even dangerous. But in the specialized world of indolent lymphomas, "watching" is actually a very deliberate, evidence-based medical strategy. It is not "doing nothing"; it is choosing the right moment to strike.

The logic behind this approach is rooted in the "indolent" nature of the disease we discussed earlier. Because follicular lymphoma often grows at a glacial pace, many people can live for years—sometimes even a decade or more—without the disease ever causing a single physical symptom or damaging an organ. If we were to start aggressive chemotherapy the moment we saw a slightly enlarged lymph node on a scan, we would be trading a patient's current high quality of life for the very real, and often permanent, side effects of treatment. Chemotherapy and even some targeted biological therapies carry risks: they can weaken the immune system, damage the bone marrow, or even increase the risk of secondary cancers later in life. If the lymphoma isn't currently bothering you, why should the treatment be allowed to?

Furthermore, there is a biological reality to consider: early treatment in follicular lymphoma has not been shown to extend a person's overall lifespan. In many other cancers, catching it early and treating it immediately is the key to survival. But because follicular lymphoma is currently viewed more like a chronic condition—think of it as "smoldering" rather than "burning"—treating it before it causes symptoms doesn't necessarily change the long-term outcome. It just means the patient spends more of their life dealing with the toxicity of medicine. By waiting, we "save" those treatments for a time when they are truly needed, ensuring that the lymphoma hasn't had as much of a chance to develop resistance to the drugs we want to use.

This period of surveillance is anything but passive. You aren't being sent away to be forgotten; you are being closely monitored through regular physical exams, blood work, and occasionally, repeat imaging. Your medical team is looking for very specific "triggers" that signal the disease is waking up. These might include a rapid increase in the size of your lymph nodes, a drop in your blood counts, or the onset of "B-symptoms" like those drenching night sweats or unexplained weight loss.

It helps to think of it like a dormant volcano. If scientists are monitoring a volcano that is merely off-gassing and not threatening any villages, they don't try to plug the crater or blow it up—that might actually make things worse. They watch the tremors, they measure the heat, and they wait. They have the equipment ready to go, but they only intervene when the data shows an eruption is actually imminent. In the same way, Active Surveillance allows you to live your life on your own terms for as long as possible, keeping the "heavy machinery" of oncology in the garage until the very moment it is required to protect your health. It is a strategy of patience, and in many cases, it is the most sophisticated and aggressive way to protect your long-term well-being.

Technical Details

The following text outlines the two most important "scoring systems" used to manage follicular lymphoma. If the previous text was about *diagnosing* the disease, this text is about *measuring* its impact and deciding *when* to start treatment.

1. The GELF Criteria: The "When to Treat" Checklist

FOLLICULAR LYMPHOMA

In follicular lymphoma, we often "Watch and Wait" because early treatment doesn't always lead to a longer life. The **GELF (Groupe d'Etude des Lymphomes de l'Folliculaire)** criteria are the industry standard used to determine if the disease has reached a "high tumor burden," meaning it's time to move from watching to active treatment.

If a patient meets **any one** of these criteria, doctors usually recommend starting therapy:

- A. **The Rule of Threes:** Having 3 or more different lymph node sites that are each 3 cm or larger.

- B. **The "Bulky" Rule:** Any single tumor mass (nodal or outside the nodes) that is 7 cm or larger.

- C. **Systemic Impact:** The presence of **B symptoms** (fever, night sweats, weight loss) or a significantly enlarged **spleen** (splenomegaly).

- D. **Fluid Buildup:** Pleural effusions (fluid around the lungs) or ascites (fluid in the abdomen) caused by the lymphoma.

- E. **Blood Count Drops (Cytopenias):** When the lymphoma invades the bone marrow so much that white blood cells drop below 1.0×10^9/L or platelets drop below 100×10^9/L.

- F. **Leukemic Phase:** When there are more than 5.0×10^9/L malignant lymphoma cells circulating in the blood.

2. FLIPI-1: The "Risk Profiler"

The **FLIPI (Follicular Lymphoma International Prognostic Index)** is a tool used at the time of diagnosis to predict how the disease is likely to behave over the long term. It doesn't necessarily tell the doctor *what* treatment to give, but it tells them how "high-risk" the case is.

You get **1 point** for each of the following risk factors:

A. **Age:** greater than or equal to 60 years.

B. **Stage:** Ann Arbor Stage III or IV (disease on both sides of the diaphragm).

C. **Hemoglobin:** Level < 12 g/dL (anemia).

D. **LDH:** Serum level above the Upper Limit of Normal (ULN).

E. **Nodal Sites:** Involvement of 5 or more distinct nodal areas.

The Risk Groups:

A. **Low Risk (0–1 factor):** Very favorable long-term outlook.

B. **Intermediate Risk (2 factors):** Moderate outlook.

C. **High Risk (greater than or equal to factors):** Indicates a more aggressive journey that may require closer monitoring or more intensive initial therapy.

These two systems work in tandem to create a personalized map. A patient might have a **High-Risk FLIPI score** (suggesting the disease is widespread), but if they don't meet any **GELF criteria** (meaning the nodes are small and they feel fine), the doctor may still choose to "Watch and Wait."

Conversely, a patient might have a **Low-Risk FLIPI**, but if they have one large 8 cm mass (meeting GELF criteria), they will likely start treatment immediately.

To see how these two systems—GELF and FLIPI—actually dictate the "vibe" of a patient's journey, it helps to look at two distinct scenarios. These demonstrate why one person might start treatment immediately while another, with seemingly more widespread disease, might be told to simply go home and enjoy their life for a while.

Scenario 1: The "High Risk" but "Low Burden" Patient

Imagine a 65-year-old man who feels perfectly fine. During a routine check-up, his doctor feels a small bump in his neck. A PET/CT scan shows tiny, 1.5 cm lymph nodes in five different areas: both sides of the neck, the armpits, and near the heart. His blood work shows a slightly elevated LDH, but his hemoglobin is normal.

    A. **FLIPI-1 Calculation:** He gets a point for **Age** (greater than or equal to 60), a point for

Stage (Stage III, since it's on both sides of the diaphragm), a point for **LDH** (above normal), and a point for **Nodal Sites** (greater than or equal to 5). His total score is **4 (High Risk)**.

B. **GELF Assessment:** He has no B symptoms (no fevers or sweats). None of his nodes are greater than or equal to cm. His blood counts are healthy, and his spleen is normal size. He meets **zero** GELF criteria.

The Outcome: Even though his FLIPI score is "High Risk," suggesting his lymphoma is widespread and biologically active, he has a **Low Tumor Burden**. Because he doesn't meet the GELF criteria, the standard of care is **Watch and Wait**. Treating him now wouldn't help him live longer; it would only give him side effects while he already feels great.

Scenario 2: The "Low Risk" but "High Burden" Patient

Now, imagine a 45-year-old woman who goes to the doctor because she has been having drenching night sweats and has a large, visible lump in her groin that makes it uncomfortable to sit. A scan shows a single, large 8 cm mass in her pelvis, but the rest of her body is completely clear. Her blood work is perfect—no anemia and a normal LDH.

A. **FLIPI-1 Calculation:** She is under 60 (0 points), Stage II because it's only in one area (0 points), normal hemoglobin (0 points), and normal LDH (0 points). She only has one nodal site (0 points). Her total score is **0 (Low Risk)**.

B. **GELF Assessment:** She has **B symptoms** (night sweats) and a **"Bulky" mass** (greater than or equal to 7 cm). She meets **two** GELF criteria.

The Outcome: Even though her FLIPI score is "Low Risk," indicating a very favorable long-term biological profile, she has a **High Tumor Burden** and significant symptoms. Because she meets the GELF criteria, she will **start treatment immediately**. Her "low risk" status is great news—it means she is likely to respond very well to therapy—but she cannot "Watch and Wait" because the disease is already interfering with her quality of life.

These scenarios show that FLIPI tells us **how the story might end** (the long-term outlook), while GELF tells us **when to start the next chapter** (when to begin treatment).

CHAPTER 7: TREATMENT OPTIONS
(THE "MENU" OF CARE)

Once you and your doctor decide that the "Watch and Wait" period has come to a close, the conversation shifts to what I like to call the "Treatment Menu." In the world of follicular lymphoma, there is no single "best" way to treat everyone. Instead, we have a series of tools, each with its own strengths, designed to be matched to the specific rhythm of your disease and the realities of your daily life. It's helpful to think of these options not as escalating steps of desperation, but as different strategies in a long-term management plan.

The foundation of almost every modern treatment is the monoclonal antibody, with rituximab being the most famous. If you recall our discussion on CD20 markers, rituximab is the precision tool designed to find those markers and stick to them. It doesn't work like traditional chemotherapy; it doesn't just kill every cell that's dividing. Instead, it "flags" the lymphoma cells so your own immune system can do the heavy lifting. Often, this is used as a standalone treatment—monotherapy—for patients who need a gentle nudge to get their disease back into a sleepy state without the side effects of stronger drugs. There is also a newer, slightly more potent version called obinutuzumab, which sticks to the cells even more tightly and can sometimes wake up the immune system more effectively in certain cases.

When the lymphoma is more active or has a higher "tumor burden," we often combine these antibodies with chemotherapy, a pairing known as chemo-immunotherapy. This is the "hammer and sniper" approach. The chemotherapy (the hammer) breaks down the bulk of the disease, while the antibody (the sniper) ensures the treatment remains targeted. You might hear acronyms like R-CHOP, R-CVP, or BR (Bendamustine-Rituximab). Bendamustine has become a favorite for many because it tends to be highly effective while being generally better tolerated than the more intensive CHOP regimen. The choice between them often comes down to a "risk versus reward" calculation: how quickly do we need a response, and how much treatment "stress" is appropriate for your body right now?

We also have "chemo-free" options that are changing the landscape, most notably the combination of rituximab and an oral drug called lenalidomide, often referred to as **R-squared (R^2)**. Lenalidomide is an immunomodulatory drug; it essentially rewires the immune environment around the lymphoma, making it much harder for the cancer cells to hide. For many, the idea of avoiding traditional IV chemotherapy while still achieving a deep, long-lasting remission is an incredibly attractive middle ground.

Then there is the category of PI3K inhibitors. A few years ago, these were the "next big thing"—oral pills that blocked a specific growth pathway inside the B-cell. However, the story of PI3K inhibitors is a cautionary tale in oncology. While they were effective at shrinking tumors, we discovered that they often came with significant side effects, like severe diarrhea or infections, and in some cases, didn't necessarily help people live longer compared to other options. Because of this, many have been withdrawn from the market or moved to a very specific "last resort" position. It's a reminder that in follicular lymphoma, more medicine isn't always better medicine; the goal is always the most effective treatment with the least amount of harm.

We are entering the era of "T-cell engagers," or bispecific antibodies like mosunetuzumab and epcoritamab. These are truly remarkable: they are engineered with two "arms"—one that grabs the lymphoma cell and one that grabs a healthy T-cell, physically dragging the two together so your immune system can't help but attack the cancer. These are currently used primarily if the disease comes back after other treatments, but they represent the future of how we might manage this chronic condition—using biology rather than poison to keep the disease at bay. The menu is long, and while that can feel overwhelming, it is actually your greatest advantage; it means if one strategy doesn't work or stops working, there is almost always another chair at another table waiting for you.

CHAPTER 8: RELAPSE AND TRANSFORMATION

One of the hardest truths to sit with after finishing treatment is that, with follicular lymphoma, the word "remission" doesn't usually mean "gone forever." Because this is a chronic, indolent condition, we view it more like a fire that has been brought down to a smolder rather than one that has been completely extinguished. For many people, that smolder stays quiet for years, or even decades. But for others, the disease eventually wakes back up. This is what we call a relapse. While the word itself sounds like a failure, in the context of this specific lymphoma, a relapse is simply a signal that it's time to change tactics. It is a known part of the journey, and the "menu" of care we discussed earlier is specifically designed with these second and third acts in mind.

However, there is a more significant shift that we always keep a watchful eye on, known as histological transformation. This is a bit different from a standard relapse. In a typical relapse, the lymphoma comes back exactly as it was before—slow-moving, Grade 1 or 2, and relatively sleepy. But in about 2% to 3% of patients each year, the follicular lymphoma cells undergo a dramatic "identity crisis." They pick up new genetic mutations that allow them to stop growing in those neat, circular follicles and start growing in a much more aggressive, "diffuse" pattern. Essentially, the indolent disease transforms into a high-grade, aggressive lymphoma, most commonly Diffuse Large B-Cell Lymphoma (DLBCL).

Think of this transformation like a houseplant that suddenly turns into a fast-growing vine that threatens to take over the room. The "indolent" rules no longer apply. This sounds frightening—and it is a serious turn in the road—but it's important to understand that a transformed lymphoma is treated very differently than a standard relapse. We move away from the "gentle" approach and toward the more intensive "hammer" treatments. Because the cells are now dividing much faster, they actually become more vulnerable to traditional, high-dose chemotherapy. The goal shifts from long-term management back to an aggressive attempt at a cure for that new, transformed component.

So, how do we know if this is happening? We don't just guess. If a patient who has been stable for years suddenly notices a single lymph node growing very rapidly, or if they start experiencing intense "B-symptoms" like drenching night sweats or a new, localized pain, we don't just assume it's a standard relapse. We usually order a PET scan. A transformed lymphoma is "hungrier" for energy than an indolent one, so it will show up much brighter on the scan. If we see a "hot spot" that looks significantly different from the others, the next step is almost always a new biopsy. We need to see the cells under the microscope to confirm if their personality has truly changed.

Dealing with the possibility of relapse or transformation requires a specific kind of mental resilience. It's about living in the "and." You are healthy *and* you have a chronic condition. You are in remission *and* you are staying vigilant. The beauty of modern oncology is that a transformed lymphoma today has a much better outlook than it did even ten years ago, thanks to new tools like CAR-T cell therapy and bispecific antibodies. Whether the disease returns as its old, sleepy self or decides to change its spots, we have a plan for both. The key is not to live in fear of the "what if," but to stay connected to your body so that if the rhythm changes, we can meet it with the right level of force at the right time.

CHAPTER 9: EMERGING FRONTIERS: CAR-T AND BISPECIFICS

As we look toward the horizon of follicular lymphoma treatment, we are moving away from the era of "carpet-bombing" the body with chemotherapy and entering a world of biological engineering. This is the realm of the "cutting edge," where the most exciting developments—CAR-T cell therapy and bispecific antibodies—are fundamentally changing what it means to live with this disease. If the treatments of the past were about poisoning the cancer, these new frontiers are about teaching the body's own immune system to be a better, more relentless hunter.

Let's start with CAR-T cell therapy, which sounds like something out of a science fiction novel but is very much a reality in the clinic today. "CAR-T" stands for Chimeric Antigen Receptor T-cell therapy. The process is remarkably personal: doctors collect your own T-cells—the "soldier" cells of your immune system—and send them to a highly specialized lab. There, scientists use genetic engineering to "reprogram" these cells, essentially giving them a new set of eyes. They add a specific receptor (the CAR) to the surface of the T-cell that is custom-built to recognize and latch onto the CD19 or CD20 protein on your lymphoma cells. Once these cells are grown into an army of millions, they are infused back into your bloodstream. They aren't just passive medicine; they are "living drugs" that circulate, multiply, and actively seek out every hidden pocket of lymphoma in the body.

While CAR-T is a powerful, one-time intensive procedure, we have another "frontier" technology that is much easier to administer but equally clever: bispecific antibodies. Think of a standard antibody as a Y-shaped molecule where both arms grab the same thing. A bispecific antibody, like mosunetuzumab or epcoritamab, is an engineered molecule where one arm grabs a lymphoma cell and the other arm grabs a healthy T-cell. In the vast, crowded space of your lymphatic system, these drugs act as a high-tech matchmaker, physically dragging the killer T-cell and the cancer cell together. By forcing this "handshake," the drug bypasses the cancer's ability to hide, essentially pointing at the lymphoma and telling the immune system, "Here is the target; do your job."

The beauty of these bispecifics is that they are often available "off-the-shelf," meaning we don't have to wait weeks to manufacture them from your own cells as we do with CAR-T. They can be given as a simple injection or infusion in a regular clinic setting. For many patients, especially those whose disease has returned after multiple other treatments, these drugs are providing deep, durable remissions that we simply didn't think were possible a decade ago. They represent a shift toward "chemo-free" living, focusing on the precision of the immune response rather than the brute force of cell-killing toxins.

Of course, these "frontier" treatments aren't without their own unique challenges. Because we are essentially supercharging the immune system, we have to watch out for things like "Cytokine Release Syndrome" (CRS), which is basically a temporary, intense inflammatory response as the T-cells go to work. It's a bit like the fever and aches you get with a bad flu, but it's a sign that the treatment is actually active. We've become very good at managing these side effects, turning what used to be a high-risk gamble into a controlled, sophisticated process. We are moving toward a future where follicular lymphoma is no longer a shadow hanging over a patient's life, but a manageable condition that can be pushed back into a long, quiet sleep by the very cells that were meant to protect us all along.

CHAPTER 10: AN ALGORITHMIC APPROACH TO TREATING FOLLICULAR LYMPHOMA

When we talk about an "algorithmic approach" to treating follicular lymphoma, it sounds like we're handing the reins over to a cold, calculating computer program. But in the hands of a seasoned oncologist, an algorithm is more like a master chef's fundamental technique—a structured way of thinking that ensures no detail is missed while allowing for the "seasoning" of individual patient needs. It is a logical flow of "if this, then that," designed to navigate the many forks in the road that this chronic disease presents over a lifetime.

The first major fork in the road appears the moment the diagnosis is confirmed. The question isn't just "What is the stage?" but rather "Does the patient need treatment today?" This is where we apply the GELF criteria, a set of benchmarks that look at the size of the lymph nodes, the impact on blood counts, and the presence of symptoms. If the "volcano" is quiet—meaning the nodes are small, the organs are happy, and the patient feels fine—the algorithm points toward active surveillance. We choose to save our ammunition. However, if the nodes are causing pain or the bone marrow is being crowded out, the algorithm shifts toward active intervention.

Once we decide to treat, the next decision point is the "first-line" strategy. For most, this involves a combination of a monoclonal antibody like rituximab and a partner therapy. If the disease is relatively mild, the partner might just be time —using rituximab alone. If the disease has more "heft," we look at adding chemotherapy, such as bendamustine or the CHOP regimen, or perhaps the "chemo-free" route with lenalidomide. This choice isn't random; it's based on a careful assessment of the patient's age, heart health, and personal goals. The goal of this first-line treatment is a "deep dive"— getting the disease as low as possible for as long as possible. If the patient achieves a good response, we then enter a "maintenance" phase, where rituximab is given every few months to keep the "brakes" on the immune system and extend the duration of that first remission.

The algorithm truly proves its worth when the disease eventually returns. This is where the map gets more complex. We first ask: "How long did that first remission last?" If the disease stayed away for more than two years (what we call POD24 negative), we can often go back to the same or similar tools with great success. But if the disease returned quickly—within 24 months—the algorithm signals that we are dealing with a more "resistant" personality. This is a critical pivot point where we move away from standard chemotherapy and toward the newer "frontier" therapies we've discussed, such as bispecific antibodies or PI3K inhibitors. We are looking to change the "biological conversation" because the previous one clearly didn't stick.

At every single relapse, the algorithm demands a "safety check" for transformation. We look at PET scans and consider a repeat biopsy to ensure the disease hasn't shifted from a slow-moving follicular lymphoma to an aggressive large-cell lymphoma. If it has transformed, the entire map changes, pointing us toward high-dose treatments and potentially a stem cell transplant or CAR-T therapy. This structured approach ensures that we are always one step ahead, anticipating the disease's next move rather than simply reacting to it. By following this logic, we provide a sense of order to what can otherwise feel like a chaotic journey, ensuring that every patient receives the right treatment, for the right reason, at the precisely right time.

Details of recommended treatment options for first-, second- and third-line therapy

This following text is the comprehensive "Playbook" for treating Follicular Lymphoma (FL). It moves from the very first treatment a patient receives to the "heavy-duty" options used if the disease comes back multiple times. The key takeaway here is that treatment is **stratified**. Doctors don't just pick a drug; they choose a path based on the "Tumor Burden" (how much lymphoma is in the body) and the patient's overall fitness.

First-Line Therapy: The Starting Blocks

If you meet the **GELF criteria** (high tumor burden), the goal is to knock the disease down effectively using a combination of an antibody and chemotherapy.

Preferred Protocols for High Tumor Burden

These regimens are used when a patient meets the **GELF criteria** (large nodes, symptoms, or impacted organ function). They almost always involve a combination of an antibody and a partner drug.

- **A. BR or BO (Bendamustine + Antibody):**
    - A. Bendamustine + **Obinutuzumab**
    - B. Bendamustine + **Rituximab**
- **B. CHOP + Antibody (Intensive Chemo):**
    - A. CHOP (Cyclophosphamide, Doxorubicin, Vincristine, Prednisone) + **Obinutuzumab**
    - B. CHOP + **Rituximab**
- **C. CVP + Antibody (Moderate Chemo):**
    - A. CVP (Cyclophosphamide, Vincristine, Prednisone) + **Obinutuzumab**
    - B. CVP + **Rituximab**
- **D. R2 (Non-Chemotherapy Immunotherapy):**
    - A. Lenalidomide + **Rituximab**

Protocols for Low Tumor Burden

These are utilized when the disease needs to be managed but hasn't reached a "bulky" or symptomatic stage.

A. Single-Agent Rituximab: Rituximab weekly for 4 doses (preferred option).

B. Alternative option: Lenalidomide + Obinutuzumab. There is clinical evidence for its use, but it is not yet the primary "gold standard" compared to the combinations listed above.

First-Line Therapy for Older or Infirm Patients

Criteria: Used if standard chemo-immunotherapy is not expected to be tolerable in the opinion of the treating physician. The preferred regimen is: **Single-Agent Rituximab; once weekly for 4 doses.**

For patients who are "infirm" (meaning they may have significant heart, kidney, or lung issues) or older patients with a lower **ECOG Performance Status**, the risks of multi-drug chemotherapy often outweigh the benefits.

A. **Gentle Mechanism:** Unlike chemotherapy, which attacks all fast-growing cells, Rituximab is a monoclonal antibody that specifically "tags" B-cells for the immune system to destroy.

B. **Avoidance of "The Hammer":** This protocol

avoids the common side effects of chemotherapy, such as severe nausea, hair loss, and the risk of life-threateningly low white blood cell counts (neutropenia).

C. **Follow-up Options:** If the patient responds well to these initial four doses, the physician may then consider "Rituximab Maintenance" (one dose every 8–12 weeks) to keep the remission going without adding toxic drugs.

Key Considerations for Selection of First-Line Therapy

When a physician chooses between these, they are typically looking at two factors:

A. **Potency vs. Toxicity:** CHOP is very effective but harder on the heart and causes hair loss; Bendamustine is often a "middle ground" in terms of side effects.

B. **Antibody Choice: Rituximab** is the reliable standard, while **Obinutuzumab** is a "Type II" antibody that can sometimes be more effective at clearing resistant cells, though it may carry a higher risk of infusion-related reactions.

Extended Therapy: "Maintenance"

After the initial "induction" phase of treatment is complete and a response has been achieved, clinical guidelines offer **First-Line Extended Therapy** (commonly known as maintenance therapy). The goal here is to prolong the remission and delay the return of the lymphoma by keeping a "patrolling" level of immunotherapy in the system.

Preferred Following Chemoimmunotherapy

These options are typically used for patients who initially had a high tumor burden and were treated with a combination of chemotherapy and an antibody (like Bendamustine, CHOP, or CVP).

A. Rituximab Maintenance (Category 1):
  A. **Dosage:** 375 mg/m^2

  B. **Schedule:** One dose every 8 to 12 weeks.

  C. **Duration:** Continued for a total of 2 years.

B. Obinutuzumab Maintenance:
  A. **Dosage:** 1 g

  B. **Schedule:** One dose every 8 weeks.

  C. **Duration:** Continued for a total of 12 doses.

Other Recommended Options

This protocol is specifically for those who received a gentler initial treatment without chemotherapy.

A. Following Single-Agent Rituximab:
  A. **Rituximab Maintenance: 375 mg/m^2**

  B. **Schedule:** One dose every 8 weeks.

  C. **Duration:** For a total of 4 doses.

Why Extended Therapy is "Optional"

While maintenance therapy significantly extends the "Progression-Free Survival" (the time the cancer stays away), it is listed as optional because it involves a trade-off.

A. **The Benefit:** It keeps the lymphoma in check for a much longer period compared to "observation" alone after induction.

B. **The Trade-off:** Long-term use of these antibodies can lead to **hypogammaglobulinemia** (low levels of healthy antibodies), which may increase the risk of recurrent infections like sinus or chest colds.

For many patients, the decision to proceed with the full two years of maintenance depends on how well they tolerated the initial treatment and their individual risk of infection.

*Second-Line and Beyond:
When the Disease Returns*

In the management of follicular lymphoma, **Second-Line Therapy** is used when the disease either doesn't respond to the initial treatment (refractory) or returns after a period of remission (relapsed). The choice of a second-line regimen depends heavily on what was used in the first round, as we generally try to avoid repeating the same "ammunition" if the disease has already found a way around it.

Preferred Regimens

These are the primary choices for patients who are fit enough for combination therapy.

- **A. Chemo-Immunotherapy Combinations:**
    - A. **Bendamustine + Obinutuzumab or Rituximab:** (Note: This is generally *not* recommended if Bendamustine was used in the first-line treatment).
    - B. **CHOP + Obinutuzumab or Rituximab:** (Cyclophosphamide, Doxorubicin, Vincristine, Prednisone).
    - C. **CVP + Obinutuzumab or Rituximab:** (Cyclophosphamide, Vincristine, Prednisone).
- **B. Targeted & Bispecific Triplets:**
    - A. **Lenalidomide + Rituximab + Epcoritamab-bysp:** A combination of an oral immune-modulator, a classic antibody, and a bispecific antibody.
    - B. **Lenalidomide + Rituximab + Tafasitamab-cxix:** Specifically for those who have had at least one prior systemic therapy.

Other Recommended Regimens

These options are often used for patients who may need a less intensive approach or for whom the preferred combinations are not suitable.

A. Immunotherapy Combinations:
  A. **Lenalidomide + Obinutuzumab or Rituximab:** (Commonly known as R2 when used with Rituximab).

B. Single-Agent Options:
  A. **Lenalidomide:** Typically reserved for those who cannot receive anti-CD20 (Rituximab/Obinutuzumab) therapy.

  B. **Obinutuzumab:** Single-agent use.

  C. **Rituximab:** Single-agent use.

Second-Line Therapy for Older or Infirm Patients

Criteria: Applied when standard combination therapies are not expected to be tolerable.

Preferred Regimens:

A. Single-Agent Rituximab:
  A. **Dosage:** 375 mg/m^2

  B. **Schedule:** Weekly for a total of 4 doses.

B. Tazemetostat:
  A. **Mechanism:** An oral pill that inhibits the EZH2 protein.

  B. **Note:** Effective regardless of whether the patient has a specific *EZH2* mutation.

Second-Line Extended Therapy (Optional)

If a patient achieves a response from their second-line treatment, these "extended" protocols are used to keep the disease in remission.

A. Rituximab Maintenance (Category 1):
   A. **Dosage:** 375 mg/m^2

   B. **Schedule:** One dose every 12 weeks.

   C. **Duration:** Continued for a total of 2 years.

B. Obinutuzumab Maintenance:
   A. **Criteria:** Specifically used if the disease is considered "rituximab-refractory" (meaning it didn't respond well to Rituximab previously).

   B. **Dosage:** 1 g

   C. **Schedule:** One dose every 8 weeks.

   D. **Duration:** For a total of 12 doses.

Why These Options Matter

This path represents a shift toward **precision medicine**.

A. **Tazemetostat** is a particularly attractive option because it is an oral medication, allowing patients to manage their treatment at home and avoid frequent clinic visits for infusions.

B. The **Rituximab 12-week schedule** is slightly

more spaced out than the standard 8-week maintenance, which can be easier for older patients to manage while still providing that "Category 1" level of proven effectiveness.

C. **Refractory Strategy:** Using **Obinutuzumab** for those who failed Rituximab is like using a more modern key for a lock that has become stuck; it targets the same CD20 marker but with a stronger "grip" on the immune system.

Key Takeaway: When moving to the second line, the oncologist's strategy is usually built on two principles:

A. **Class Switching:** If the lymphoma grew through Bendamustine, switching to a regimen like **CHOP** or the **Lenalidomide** triplets is vital because it attacks the cancer cells via a different biological pathway.

B. **The "POD24" Factor:** If the disease returns very quickly (within 24 months of the first treatment), it is considered more aggressive, and the doctor may lean toward the newer, more potent combinations involving bispecific antibodies like **Epcoritamab**.

In the management of relapsed or refractory follicular lymphoma, the priority for patients who are older or physically "infirm" is to provide effective disease control while strictly avoiding the severe side effects of intensive chemotherapy. These protocols focus on targeted therapies that are generally better tolerated.

Third-Line and "The Frontiers":
The Big Guns

When we reach the stage of **Third-Line and Subsequent Therapy**, the clinical strategy shifts toward some of the most innovative and potent tools in modern medicine. At this point, the lymphoma has likely shown it can bypass traditional chemotherapy and first-generation immunotherapies. Consequently, the focus turns to "re-educating" your own immune system or using highly specific molecular keys to unlock the cancer's defenses.

It is also important to note that any **Second-Line** regimens that weren't used previously remain valid options here. However, the "preferred" choices in the third line represent a significant leap in technology.

Preferred: T-Cell Mediated Therapies

These treatments are designed to take the "brakes" off your immune system or physically force your healthy T-cells to attack the lymphoma.

- A. **Bispecific Antibody Therapy:** These drugs act like a biological "matchmaker," with one arm that grabs the lymphoma cell and another that grabs a healthy T-cell, pulling them together so the T-cell can destroy the cancer.

A. Epcoritamab-bysp

   B. Mosunetuzumab-axgb

B. **Chimeric Antigen Receptor (CAR) T-Cell Therapy:** This is a sophisticated "living drug." Your T-cells are collected, genetically engineered in a lab to recognize the **CD19** protein on lymphoma cells, and kemudian re-infused into your body.

   A. Axicabtagene ciloleucel

   B. Lisocabtagene maraleucel

   C. Tisagenlecleucel

Other Recommended Targeted Therapies

For patients who may not be candidates for the intensive nature of CAR-T or who prefer a different biological approach, several targeted "non-chemo" options are available.

   A. **EZH2 Inhibitor: Tazemetostat** (effective regardless of mutation status).

   B. **BTK Inhibitor (BTKi): Zanubrutinib** combined with **Obinutuzumab**. This targets a specific signaling pathway (Bruton's Tyrosine Kinase) that B-cells use to grow.

   C. **Antibody-Drug Conjugate: Loncastuximab tesirine-lpyl** combined with **Rituximab** (Category 2B). This acts like a "Trojan Horse," delivering a potent toxin directly inside the B-cell.

Third-Line Consolidation Therapy

Consolidation is about "locking in" a remission. While less common than it used to be due to the success of CAR-T and bispecifics, it remains a powerful tool in specific cases. **Allogeneic Hematopoietic Cell Transplantation (HCT)** is the therapy of choice here. This involves replacing your entire immune system with that of a healthy donor. It is considered "useful in certain circumstances," particularly for younger, fit patients with very aggressive or frequently recurring disease.

Key Takeaway: If one path doesn't work, there are multiple "biological backdoors" we can now use to target follicular lymphoma cells.

Notes on Response Criteria

The **Lugano Response Criteria** are essentially the "universal grading system" used by oncologists to determine how well a treatment is working. When you finish a cycle of chemotherapy or reach the end of a treatment plan, the doctors need a standardized way to say whether the lymphoma is gone, shrinking, or staying the same.

The criteria look at two things simultaneously: **Radiologic response** (how big the nodes look on a CT) and **Metabolic response** (how "bright" or active they look on a PET scan).

The 5-Point Scale (The "Deauville" Scale)

One of the most important parts of this text is the **5-Point Scale (5-PS)**. It's a way to measure the PET scan's "brightness" by comparing the lymphoma sites to parts of your body that naturally glow on a scan (the mediastinum/chest and the liver).

A. **Score 1:** No uptake (the area is "dark").

B. **Score 2:** Uptake is less than or equal to the chest area (mediastinum).

C. **Score 3:** Uptake is slightly higher than the chest but less than or equal to the liver.

D. **Score 4:** Uptake is moderately higher than the liver.

E. **Score 5:** Uptake is markedly higher than the liver or new spots have appeared.

Note that **Scores 1, 2, and 3** are considered a **Complete Metabolic Response**.

Understanding the Response Categories

The text breaks the results down into four specific "grades" on your report card:

A. Complete Response (CR) — The "All Clear"

A. This is the goal of treatment.

B. **On PET:** You score a 1, 2, or 3. Even if a mass is still visible on the CT, if it isn't "glowing" on the PET, it's considered dead tissue or scarring.

- C. **On CT:** All target lymph nodes must shrink to less than or equal to 1.5 cm.
- D. **Bone Marrow:** If the marrow was involved before, it must now be clear.

B. **Partial Response (PR) — "Significant Progress"**
- A. The treatment is working, but the disease isn't entirely gone.
- B. **On PET:** You score a 4 or 5, but the "brightness" is lower than it was at the start of treatment.
- C. **On CT:** There is a greater than or equal to 50% decrease in the size of the lymph nodes (measured by the "Sum of the Product of Diameters" or SPD).

C. **No Response / Stable Disease (SD) — "Treading Water"**
- A. The disease hasn't gotten significantly better, but it hasn't gotten worse either.
- B. **On PET:** You score a 4 or 5 with no real change in the brightness.
- C. **On CT:** There is less than a 50% decrease in size, but no evidence of growth or new lesions.

D. **Progressive Disease (PD) — "Getting Worse"**
- A. This indicates that the current treatment is no longer controlling the lymphoma.

B. **On PET:** The score is 4 or 5, and the intensity has increased, or entirely new "hot spots" have appeared.

   C. **On CT:** At least one node has grown significantly (by 50% or more) or new nodes larger than 1.5 cm have appeared.

Why we use both PET and CT

PET-CT is the gold standard for most lymphomas because it tells us if the cells are *alive*, not just how big they are. However, for some very slow-growing types, a standard CT is often enough because those cells don't always "glow" brightly on a PET scan.

A Note on "False Positives"

The criteria include a warning: **not everything that glows is cancer.** Infection or inflammation (like after a flu shot or a cold) can cause a "Score 4 or 5." If a scan shows a new spot but you feel fine, the "gold standard" is still a biopsy to confirm it's actually the lymphoma returning.

CHAPTER 11: THE LYMPHOMA-FRIENDLY KITCHEN

In the world of follicular lymphoma, the kitchen often becomes your most important pharmacy. While the medical team manages the infusions and the scans, what happens at your dining table is the work you do every day to support your body's resilience. It isn't about following a restrictive "cancer diet" or chasing miracle cures in a blender; it's about creating an environment—an internal ecosystem—that is as hostile to inflammation as possible while giving your healthy cells the fuel they need to keep standing.

The cornerstone of this approach is anti-inflammatory eating. If you think of inflammation as a low-grade fire smoldering in the background of a chronic condition like lymphoma, your food choices can either be the water or the gasoline. You want to lean heavily into the "water" category: vibrant, colorful vegetables, leafy greens, and the deep blues and reds of berries, which are packed with antioxidants that act like a cleanup crew for cellular damage. Incorporating healthy fats, like those found in walnuts, flaxseeds, and fatty fish, provides your body with omega-3s—the natural "anti-freeze" for systemic inflammation. Even your spice cabinet holds power; a pinch of turmeric or a grate of fresh ginger isn't just for flavor; they are potent, natural tools that have been used for centuries to quiet the body's inflammatory pathways.

However, the reality of treatment often brings a specific challenge: steroids. Whether it's dexamethasone or prednisone, these drugs are vital for managing the lymphoma, but they can be a "wolf in sheep's clothing" when it comes to your metabolism. They trick your brain into feeling a ravenous, bottomless hunger and can cause your body to hold onto water and salt, leading to that characteristic "moon face" or weight gain around the midsection. The trick to managing this isn't through willpower alone—it's through strategy. To combat the fluid retention, try to dial down the salt and dial up the potassium. Foods like bananas, kiwis, and avocados help balance out the sodium, encouraging your body to let go of that extra water weight. To manage the "steroid hunger," focus on high-protein snacks and fiber-rich whole grains like oats or lentils. These take longer to digest, keeping you feeling full and preventing the blood sugar spikes that steroids often trigger.

Then there is the quiet, often overlooked hero of the journey: hydration. When you are undergoing treatment, your kidneys and liver are working overtime to process medications and flush out the byproducts of broken-down lymphoma cells. Water is the solvent that keeps this machinery moving.

If plain water starts to taste metallic—a common side effect of some therapies—don't force it. Get creative. Infuse your water with slices of cucumber, a sprig of mint, or a few frozen berries to make it more palatable. You can also "eat" your hydration; watermelon, cucumbers, and even simple vegetable broths are mostly water and can be much easier to stomach on days when you're feeling a bit of "treatment fatigue."

The goal of a lymphoma-friendly kitchen is to take some of the power back. It's about recognizing that while you may not have control over the genetic "glitches" in your B-cells, you do have control over what you put on your plate. By eating with intention —prioritizing protein to protect your muscles, using spices to fight inflammation, and staying hydrated to flush the system—you are doing the vital, daily work of a survivor. It's a slow, steady process of nourishing yourself back to strength, one meal at a time.

CHAPTER 12: MOVEMENT AS MEDICINE

In the journey of managing follicular lymphoma, exercise is often the most underutilized tool in our kit. We tend to think of movement as something we do when we are healthy, a reward for feeling good, but in the context of a chronic condition, movement actually becomes the medicine that helps us *get* healthy. It isn't about training for a marathon or hitting personal records in the gym; it's about maintaining the integrity of your body's systems so they can better handle the stress of the disease and its treatments.

During the "Watch and Wait" phase, your goal is essentially "pre-habilitation." You have the gift of time and, usually, a relatively stable level of energy. This is the moment to build a physical reserve. Think of your body like a battery; the stronger and more efficient your muscles and cardiovascular system are now, the longer you can "run" if you eventually face more intensive therapy. A balanced mix of moderate aerobic activity—like brisk walking or cycling—and light resistance training is ideal. Strength training is particularly important here because it helps maintain bone density and muscle mass, both of which can be challenged later by medications like steroids. The goal isn't intensity; it's consistency. You're essentially "armoring" your body for the future.

When you move into the active treatment phase, such as chemotherapy, the philosophy of movement has to shift. This is the time for "maintenance and management." You will likely face days where the fatigue feels like a heavy wool blanket, making even the walk to the kitchen feel like an expedition. The instinct is to stay in bed, but total rest can actually worsen "cancer-related fatigue." The secret is to keep the "engine" idling. Even on your hardest days, gentle stretching or a five-minute stroll around the house can prevent your joints from stiffening and keep your circulation moving. It sends a signal to your nervous system that you are still in control. On the days you feel better, you can do more, but the golden rule during chemo is to listen to your body's "check engine" light. If you're exhausted, scale back to gentle yoga or breath-focused movement. You aren't trying to build new muscle right now; you're simply trying to keep what you have.

Recovery is perhaps the most rewarding phase, but it requires the most patience. Once the infusions stop, there is often a rush of "I want my life back" energy, but the body usually recovers in waves rather than a straight line. Your immune system and your bone marrow have been through a significant event, and your "battery" might still be prone to draining quickly. This is the time for a gradual "re-entry." Start with low-impact activities—swimming is excellent because it's easy on the joints—and slowly increase your duration before you increase your intensity. It's about rebuilding your "baseline." Pay close attention to your balance and flexibility, as some treatments can cause minor peripheral neuropathy (numbness in the feet), which makes steady, mindful movement even more important for safety.

Movement as medicine is about reclaiming your agency. Lymphoma can make you feel like your body has betrayed you, but when you choose to move—even if it's just a ten-minute walk—you are asserting your own power. You are telling your body that it is more than just a host for a diagnosis; it is a living, breathing, capable vessel. Whether you are in a quiet "watchful" period or the thick of recovery, remember that the best exercise is the one you actually do. It doesn't have to be perfect; it just has to be yours.

CHAPTER 13: THE ART OF RESTORATIVE SLEEP

When we talk about recovering from follicular lymphoma, we often focus on the "active" parts—the infusions, the diet, the exercise. But there is a silent, foundational pillar that holds everything else up, and that is sleep. In the context of lymphoma, sleep isn't just "down time"; it is the period when your bone marrow does its most intensive construction work and your immune system recalibrates. Yet, ironically, a diagnosis of lymphoma often brings with it a perfect storm of sleep disturbances. Between the "scanxiety" that keeps your mind racing at 3:00 AM, the physical discomfort of enlarged nodes, and the chemical interference of medications like steroids, the simple act of falling asleep can start to feel like a lost art.

To reclaim your rest, you first have to understand the specific hurdles in your way. For many, the biggest culprit is the "steroid surge." If you are on a regimen that includes prednisone or dexamethasone, these drugs essentially mimic the body's natural stress hormones. They put you in a state of high alert, making your brain feel wired even when your muscles are exhausted. If this is your reality, timing is everything. Whenever possible, talk to your team about taking these medications as early in the morning as allowed. By doing so, you give the drug's "caffeine-like" peak a chance to wear off before your head hits the pillow. It's about working with the medication's rhythm rather than fighting against it.

Then there is the physical environment. Lymphoma can sometimes cause night sweats—those drenching episodes that force you to wake up and change your sheets. This isn't just a nuisance; it's a major disruptor of deep, restorative REM sleep. Managing this requires a bit of "sleep engineering." Switch to moisture-wicking fabrics rather than heavy cotton, and consider a "layered" bedding approach so you can adjust your temperature quickly without fully waking up. Keeping a spare set of pajamas and a towel on the nightstand can also shorten the "awake time" if a sweat does occur, allowing you to slide back into sleep before your brain fully clicks into "daytime mode."

Beyond the physical, we have to address the "mental chatter." Living with a chronic condition creates a specific kind of cognitive load. Your brain, in an attempt to protect you, spends the quiet hours of the night scanning for threats—worrying about blood counts or the next appointment. To counter this, you need a "buffer zone" between your day and your sleep. This isn't just about turning off the TV; it's about a deliberate ritual that signals safety to your nervous system. Whether it's five minutes of box breathing—inhaling, holding, and exhaling to equal counts—or a "brain dump" where you write down every worry on a physical piece of paper to deal with tomorrow, these practices act as an "off-switch" for the sympathetic nervous system.

Try to view sleep as a skill rather than a given. If you can't sleep after twenty minutes, don't stay in bed and associate your mattress with frustration. Get up, keep the lights low, and do something monotonous—like folding socks or reading a book you've already finished—until the "sleep wave" returns. By treating your rest with the same respect and strategy as your medical treatments, you transform your bedroom from a place of midnight worry into a sanctuary of healing. Sleep is the bridge that carries you from the fatigue of today to the strength of tomorrow, and learning to cross it reliably is one of the most powerful things you can do for your long-term health.

CHAPTER 14: NEUTROPENIC LIVING: STAYING SAFE IN A GERM-FILLED WORLD

Living with neutropenia—a state where your primary defense force of white blood cells, the neutrophils, is significantly thinned out—can feel like being a castle with its outer walls temporarily dismantled. In a healthy state, your immune system is a silent, efficient screening process that handles millions of germs every day without you even noticing. When you are neutropenic, however, that screening process is on hiatus. The world doesn't become more dangerous, but your ability to navigate it changes. The goal of "neutropenic living" isn't to retreat into a bubble, but to develop a sophisticated, second-nature habit of hygiene that allows you to live your life while keeping the germs at arm's length.

The kitchen is your first and most important frontline. In a normal immune environment, a slightly undercooked egg or a piece of unwashed fruit is rarely a problem. When your neutrophil count is low, these become potential entry points for bacteria. The rule of thumb here is "heat is your friend." Cooking food thoroughly—until it is piping hot all the way through—kills the vast majority of the pathogens that your body would otherwise have to fight. This means saying a temporary goodbye to sushi, rare steaks, and "sunny-side up" eggs with runny yolks. You should also be wary of the deli counter and open buffets. These are "communal" food spaces where cross-contamination is almost impossible to control. Stick to freshly prepared meals at home, and when you do buy produce, wash it with the kind of focus a surgeon uses before a procedure. Even thick-skinned fruits like oranges or melons should be scrubbed before they are cut, as the knife can carry bacteria from the outside skin right into the heart of the fruit.

Then there is the question of the outside world and the crowds that come with it. You don't have to become a hermit, but you do have to become a strategist. "Off-peak" living is the secret to staying social without the risk. If you need to go to the grocery store or a pharmacy, try to go during the quietest hours of the Tuesday morning rather than the Saturday afternoon rush. When it comes to masking, don't view it as a symbol of illness, but as a high-tech filter for your "castle gates." A well-fitted N95 or surgical mask in a crowded indoor space significantly reduces your exposure to respiratory viruses that could turn into a serious complication when your counts are low. If a friend or family member has even a "slight tickle" in their throat or a minor cold, it is perfectly okay—and medically necessary—to ask them to visit another time. True friends will understand that your safety is the priority.

For many of us, our pets are a vital source of emotional comfort, and the good news is that you don't have to give up that bond. However, you do need to rethink how you interact with them. Pets can carry bacteria and parasites that are harmless to them but problematic for you. The most important rule is to delegate the "dirty work." Someone else should be responsible for cleaning the cat's litter box, picking up after the dog, or cleaning the birdcage. If you must handle these tasks, wear gloves and a mask, and wash your hands immediately afterward. Avoid "rough play" that could lead to scratches or bites, as even a small break in the skin can become an infection site. And while it's tempting to let your dog give you "kisses," try to keep their affection away from your face and mouth. A quick handwash after a petting session is a small price to pay for the immense mental health benefits of having your companion by your side.

The most powerful tool in your arsenal is the simplest: handwashing. It sounds basic, but 20 seconds of scrubbing with warm, soapy water is the single most effective way to break the chain of infection. Get into the habit of washing your hands every time you come home, before you eat, and after you touch high-traffic surfaces like doorknobs or remote controls. And finally, remember the "Red Alert" rule: in a neutropenic state, a fever is not just a symptom; it is a medical emergency. If your temperature hits 100.4°F (38°C) or higher, your "castle" is calling for reinforcements. Don't wait until the morning to see if it goes away. Call your oncology team immediately. This vigilance, combined with smart daily habits, is what allows you to move through the world with confidence, knowing that you are actively protecting your recovery every step of the way.

CHAPTER 15: INTEGRATIVE THERAPIES: BEYOND THE PRESCRIPTION

In the journey of managing a condition like follicular lymphoma, there is a tendency to focus entirely on the "high-tech" side of things—the targeted antibodies, the genetic markers, and the complex treatment algorithms. But for many, the most profound improvements in quality of life come from what we call integrative therapies. This isn't about "alternative" medicine that tries to replace your oncologist's plan; rather, it is about "integrative" care that works alongside it. Think of your medical treatment as the force that targets the cancer, while integrative therapies like yoga, acupuncture, and meditation are the tools that support the *person* living within that body. They help manage the "collateral damage" of the disease—the stress, the fatigue, and the physical discomfort that even the best drugs can't always reach.

Yoga is perhaps the most well-studied of these practices in the cancer setting. When you move through a gentle yoga sequence, you aren't just stretching your muscles; you are engaging in a sophisticated conversation with your nervous system. Many patients find that the deep, rhythmic breathing of yoga helps move the body out of a state of "fight or flight"—that high-alert stress mode we often live in after a diagnosis—and into a state of "rest and digest." The science backs this up, showing that regular, gentle yoga can significantly reduce the "cancer-related fatigue" that often feels so heavy and immovable. It helps maintain the flexibility of the lymphatic system itself, encouraging the fluid to flow more freely through the very nodes we are keeping such a close eye on. It's a way of reclaiming your body, reminding yourself that it is a place of movement and strength, not just a site for medical procedures.

Then there is the ancient practice of acupuncture. For someone used to the precision of modern needles in a hospital setting, the idea of tiny, hair-thin needles being placed along "meridians" can feel a bit abstract. However, the biological evidence is increasingly clear. We now know that acupuncture stimulates the nervous system to release natural chemicals—like endorphins and enkephalins—that alter how our brain perceives pain. In the world of lymphoma, acupuncture is frequently used to manage the nausea that can follow treatment or the "pins and needles" sensation of peripheral neuropathy that some medications cause. It doesn't just mask the symptom; it seems to help "reset" the signaling pathways that have been disrupted. It's a subtle but powerful way to dial down the volume on the body's distress signals.

Perhaps the most accessible, yet most challenging, of these tools is meditation and mindfulness. When you receive a diagnosis of a chronic condition, your mind often becomes a time traveler—constantly rushing into the future to worry about the next scan or retreating into the past to wonder what went wrong. Meditation is the practice of tethering yourself to the only moment you actually have: right now. Whether it's a guided visualization or simply focusing on the sensation of your breath, meditation has been shown to lower levels of cortisol, the body's primary stress hormone. By lowering cortisol, you aren't just "feeling better" emotionally; you are creating a more stable internal environment where your immune system can function more efficiently. It is the art of finding a "quiet room" inside your own mind, regardless of how chaotic the medical news might feel on the outside.

These therapies are about wholeness. They remind us that healing is not just about the absence of disease, but the presence of well-being. They provide a sense of agency in a process that can often feel like it's out of your hands. Whether you are in a period of "Watch and Wait" or in the middle of active recovery, incorporating these practices isn't a luxury; it is a vital part of your maintenance plan. They help you build the resilience needed to face the marathons, ensuring that while the medicine takes care of the cells, you are taking care of the soul.

CHAPTER 16: CRACKING THE CODE OF CANCER FATIGUE

In the world of follicular lymphoma, there is a specific type of exhaustion that goes far beyond being "tired." It's a heavy, bone-deep weariness that doesn't disappear with a good night's sleep or an extra cup of coffee. We call it cancer-related fatigue, and for many, it is the most disruptive part of the entire experience. To manage it, you have to stop thinking of your energy as an infinite resource and start thinking of it as a daily currency. This is where the "Spoon Theory" comes in—a simple but profound analogy that helps patients and their families understand the hidden economy of living with a chronic illness.

Imagine that every morning you wake up with exactly twelve spoons. Each task you perform throughout the day costs you a spoon. Getting dressed might cost one; making a meal might cost two; a focused conversation with a friend could cost another. In a healthy state, you have an unlimited supply of spoons, so you never have to count them. But when your body is diverted by lymphoma—either fighting the disease itself or repairing the "collateral damage" from treatment—your drawer of spoons is suddenly very small. If you use all twelve spoons by lunchtime, you are essentially "bankrupt" for the rest of the day. There is no overdraft protection; once the energy is gone, the wall hits.

Cracking the code of this fatigue requires you to become an expert in energy conservation. This doesn't mean you stop living; it means you become highly intentional about how you spend your limited currency. We often talk about the "Four Ps": Planning, Pacing, Prioritizing, and Positioning. Planning means looking at your week and realizing that if you have a doctor's appointment on Tuesday, you probably shouldn't schedule a grocery trip for Wednesday. Pacing is the art of breaking a large task—like cleaning a room—into three smaller tasks with rest breaks in between. You aren't being lazy; you're being strategic. You're ensuring that you don't use three spoons on a task that could have cost one if you'd just taken your time.

Prioritizing is perhaps the hardest part, because it requires saying "no" to things you feel you *should* do so that you have the energy for things you *want* to do. It's okay to let the laundry sit for another day if it means you have the energy to read a story to your son or sit in the garden for an hour. Positioning is a more literal strategy—it's about changing how you do things to save physical effort. Sitting on a stool while you prep dinner or using a rolling cart to move items around the house might seem like small changes, but they are the "cents" that add up to a full spoon by the end of the day.

It's also vital to understand that this fatigue isn't just physical; it's often cognitive. We call it "chemobrain" or "brain fog," and it's essentially the mental equivalent of a low battery. When your brain is tired, processing complex information or making decisions feels like wading through knee-deep mud. During these times, give yourself permission to use "external brains." Use the notes app on your phone, set alarms for everything, and don't be afraid to ask people to repeat themselves. By offloading the mental work to these tools, you preserve more of your "mental spoons" for the things that actually matter.

Managing cancer fatigue is about self-compassion. It is about acknowledging that your body is currently doing the incredible, invisible work of healing. You wouldn't expect a marathon runner to mow the lawn immediately after a race; your body is running a marathon every single day. By using the Spoon Theory to explain your needs to your family and using energy conservation to protect your daily currency, you shift the power dynamic. The fatigue may be a persistent houseguest, but with the right strategies, you can ensure it doesn't get to decide how you spend your most precious moments.

CHAPTER 17: MANAGING THE "QUEASIES": NAUSEA & DIGESTIVE HEALTH

One of the most universal anxieties when facing lymphoma treatment is the fear of nausea—that lingering, unsettled feeling often referred to as "the queasies." While modern medicine has made incredible strides in preventing the severe vomiting that once defined the chemotherapy experience, many patients still navigate a subtle, persistent digestive "off-ness." It can feel like being permanently seasick, where your favorite foods suddenly smell wrong and the very idea of a full meal feels overwhelming. Managing this isn't just about the pills your doctor prescribes; it's about a broader, more intuitive approach to digestive health that starts with how you eat and how you listen to your body's signals.

The first strategy for calming a rebellious stomach is to rethink the traditional "three square meals" structure. When your digestive system is stressed by treatment or the disease itself, a large plate of food can feel like a mountain you're being asked to climb. Instead, aim for the "nibble and sip" method. Small, frequent snacks throughout the day keep your stomach from ever being completely empty, which, counterintuitively, is often when nausea is at its worst. Think of your stomach like a gentle fire;

you want to keep adding small twigs of fuel rather than dumping a heavy log on it all at once.

What you choose to nibble on matters just as much as how often you do it. During the peak days of treatment, the "bland is best" rule usually wins. We often recommend the BRAT diet—bananas, rice, applesauce, and toast—because these foods are incredibly easy for the gut to break down and don't have strong aromas that might trigger a wave of queasiness. Cold or room-temperature foods are also secret weapons in your arsenal. Hot foods release more steam, and that steam carries concentrated smells that can be overwhelming. A chilled pasta salad, a turkey wrap, or even a simple fruit smoothie can be much more approachable than a steaming bowl of soup or a hot roast.

Beyond the food itself, there are powerful non-drug remedies that have stood the test of time. Ginger is perhaps the most famous, and for good reason. It contains compounds called gingerols that help speed up the "emptying" of the stomach, preventing food from sitting too long and causing that heavy, nauseated feeling. Whether it's real ginger ale (look for brands with actual ginger root), ginger tea, or even crystallized ginger chews, it acts as a natural "pacifier" for the digestive tract. Peppermint is another classic ally; the menthol in peppermint oil helps relax the muscles of the stomach and improves the flow of bile, which the body uses to digest fats. A simple cup of peppermint tea or even sniffing a bit of peppermint essential oil can sometimes break a spell of nausea in minutes.

We also shouldn't overlook the "mechanical" side of digestion. For example, staying upright for at least an hour after eating allows gravity to help your stomach do its job, reducing the risk of acid reflux or that "stuck" feeling. Some patients also find incredible relief using acupressure bands—those simple elastic wristbands with a plastic stud that presses on the P6 point, located just above the wrist. While it might seem overly simple, this pressure point is a well-recognized gateway to the nervous system's nausea-control center, providing a constant, drug-free "signal" of calm to the brain.

Managing your digestive health during this journey is about moving from a place of frustration to one of curiosity. Every patient has a unique "safe list" of foods and rituals that work for them. By keeping the portions small, opting for cool and bland choices, and leaning on natural wonders like ginger and acupressure, you take the edge off the "queasies." You aren't just enduring a side effect; you are actively soothing your system, ensuring that your body remains a well-nourished vessel for the healing work it is doing every day.

CHAPTER 18: THE FOG: COPING WITH "CHEMO BRAIN"

For many people navigating follicular lymphoma, the most frustrating side effect isn't something they can see on a scan or feel in a lymph node. It's a subtle, frustrating cloudiness that drifts over the mind, often called "chemo brain" or, more accurately, cancer-related cognitive impairment. It's the feeling of walking into a room and having no idea why you're there, or searching for a common word that feels like it's just behind a heavy curtain. If your brain was once a high-speed fiber-optic connection, chemo brain can make it feel like you're back on dial-up. It isn't just a product of the drugs themselves; it's a combination of the body's inflammatory response, the stress of the diagnosis, and the mental exhaustion of managing a chronic condition.

The first step in coping with this fog is to stop fighting against it and start working around it. Think of your brain's processing power right now as a finite battery. In the past, you could run dozens of "apps" in the background—remembering birthdays, planning dinner, and managing a work project all at once. Now, you need to "force quit" those background tasks to save energy for the thing right in front of you. This is where organizational tools become your external hard drive. Don't rely on your internal memory for anything that can be written down. Whether it's a physical notebook you carry everywhere or a robust notes app on your phone, getting the information out of your head and onto a page immediately lowers your cognitive load. If it's written down, your brain doesn't have to keep "pinging" that memory to make sure it's still there.

Beyond just staying organized, you can actually engage in "physical therapy" for your mind. Cognitive exercises aren't about becoming a grandmaster at chess; they are about keeping the neural pathways flexible. This could be as simple as changing your routine—brushing your teeth with your non-dominant hand or taking a new route to the grocery store. These small shifts force the brain to forge new connections. Word puzzles, Sudoku, or even learning a few phrases in a new language can help, but the key is to keep it enjoyable. If a puzzle makes you feel stressed or defeated, it's counterproductive. You want "gentle resistance" training for the mind, not a grueling exam.

We also have to talk about the physical environment of the brain. Your neurons are incredibly sensitive to what's happening in the rest of your body. If you are dehydrated, the fog will be thicker. If you haven't slept well—as we discussed in the art of restorative sleep—the "trash" that builds up in your brain overnight doesn't get cleared out, leading to more cloudiness the next day. Even mild exercise, like a short walk, can help by increasing blood flow and oxygen to the brain. Think of it as opening a window in a stuffy room; it doesn't solve everything, but it certainly helps the air clear faster.

Give yourself the grace of the "single-tasking" rule. Multitasking is a myth even for the healthiest people, but for someone dealing with chemo brain, it's a recipe for burnout. If you are on the phone, don't try to check your email. If you are cooking, don't try to listen to a complex podcast. Focus on the one thing you are doing, finish it, and then move to the next. By narrowing your focus, you reduce the chances of a "system crash."

It's important to remember that for the vast majority of people, this fog is temporary. It's a side effect of a body under siege, and as your system recovers and the inflammation settles, the "dial-up" speed eventually returns to broadband. In the meantime, use your tools, lean on your "external brain," and be patient with yourself. You are still in there; the signal is just a little noisy right now.

CHAPTER 19: TAMING THE FIRE: NEUROPATHY & NERVE PAIN

One of the more jarring side effects of certain lymphoma treatments is the sensation that your nervous system has developed a mind of its own. We call it peripheral neuropathy, but for many, it feels like a bizarre internal weather system—alternating between a pins-and-needles tingling, a sudden electric jolt, or a strange, heavy numbness in the hands and feet. This happens because some of our most effective therapies can be a bit "over-zealous"; while they are excellent at targeting the lymphoma, they can sometimes singe the protective coating of the long, delicate nerves that reach out to your fingers and toes. It's like having a frayed electrical cord in your house; the power is still there, but the signal is erratic and prone to sparking.

When your nerves aren't sending accurate messages to your brain, your world becomes a bit more unpredictable, which makes home safety a top priority. Numbness is particularly deceptive because it removes your body's natural early-warning system. You might not realize a bath is scalding hot or that a shoe is rubbing a blister until the damage is already done. To manage this, you have to replace your "feeling" with "seeing." Get into the habit of checking the temperature of water with an elbow or a thermometer rather than a hand. Inspect your feet every night with a small mirror, looking for any redness or breaks in the skin that you might not have felt. It's about becoming a vigilant observer of your own body, ensuring that a lack of sensation doesn't lead to a lack of care.

The environment around you needs a bit of "nerve-proofing" as well. Because neuropathy can affect your balance and your sense of where your feet are in space—what we call proprioception—the risk of a trip or fall becomes much higher. This is the time to be ruthless with your home decor. Clear away the "tripping hazards": the loose area rugs, the tangled extension cords, and the low-profile coffee tables. Improving the lighting in hallways and bathrooms is essential, especially for those midnight trips when your brain is already a bit foggy. Think of it as creating a "clear runway" for yourself; the fewer obstacles your feet have to navigate, the more confident you will feel moving through your day.

When it comes to the actual discomfort—the burning or the tingling—there are ways to "quiet the fire" without always reaching for a prescription bottle. While there are certainly medications that can help dampen nerve pain, many patients find relief through temperature and texture. For some, lukewarm soaks with Epsom salts can soothe the "electric" feeling, while others find that keeping their hands and feet cool is the key. You might also explore "desensitization" techniques, which involve gently rubbing different textures—like a soft silk scarf followed by a slightly rougher washcloth—over the affected areas. This helps "retrain" the nerves, teaching them to distinguish between normal touch and a pain signal.

It's also worth noting that movement, as counterintuitive as it feels when your feet hurt, is one of your best allies. Gentle exercise keeps the blood flowing to those distant nerve endings, providing them with the oxygen and nutrients they need to attempt repairs. Even while sitting, simple ankle circles or "scrunching" a towel with your toes can keep the "signal" alive. Be patient with this process; nerves are the slow-growers of the human body. They don't heal overnight, but with a combination of safety habits, gentle stimulation, and a bit of environmental adjustment, you can turn down the volume on the "nerve noise" and reclaim your sense of stability.

CHAPTER 20: SKIN, HAIR, AND NAILS: THE EXTERNAL JOURNEY

While so much of the conversation around follicular lymphoma focuses on what's happening deep inside the lymph nodes or the bone marrow, the reality is that the journey often leaves its most visible marks on the surface—our skin, hair, and nails. These are our "external frontiers," and because many of our most effective treatments are designed to target rapidly dividing cells or specific immune markers, these visible parts of us often get caught in the crossfire. It can feel like a secondary burden to look in the mirror and see a different version of yourself, but understanding the "why" behind these changes and having a toolkit to manage them can help you feel more in control of your own reflection.

One of the most common external side effects is what we often call the "Rituximab Rash." Because Rituximab is a monoclonal antibody that wakes up the immune system, your body can sometimes get a little over-enthusiastic, manifesting as a red, itchy, or bumpy rash, often on the face, chest, or back. It isn't an "allergy" in the traditional sense; it's more of an inflammatory "hello" from your immune system as it processes the medication. The key here is to be as gentle as possible. This isn't the time for harsh exfoliating scrubs or scented "anti-acne" washes. Think of your skin as a piece of delicate silk that has been through a storm. Use lukewarm water, soap-free cleansers, and thick, fragrance-free moisturizers that contain ceramides to help rebuild the skin's natural barrier. If the rash becomes truly uncomfortable or "hot," a cool compress or a doctor-approved hydrocortisone cream can help turn down the heat.

When it comes to hair, follicular lymphoma treatment is usually a different story than the total hair loss we often associate with "Hollywood" chemotherapy. While some intensive regimens might cause significant loss, many of the more modern, targeted therapies lead to what we call "thinning" or "shedding." It can feel like your hair has simply lost its "spark" or volume. This happens because the hair follicles enter a resting phase to conserve energy for the body's healing process. To manage this, less is definitely more. Avoid high-heat styling tools like flat irons or blow dryers, which can make fragile hair more prone to breakage. Switch to a wide-tooth comb and consider a "no-pressure" hairstyle. It's also a good time to pamper your scalp —gentle massages can improve circulation to the follicles, and using a silk pillowcase can reduce the friction that leads to tangling and pulling during the night.

Your nails, too, might join the journey, becoming brittle, developing ridges, or even changing color slightly. Nails are essentially a "history log" of your health; every time you have a treatment infusion, it creates a tiny "speed bump" in the growth of the nail. To protect them, keep them trimmed short to prevent snagging and use a heavy-duty cuticle oil or plain petroleum jelly several times a day. If you're a fan of manicures, try to avoid the "gel" or "acrylic" types that require soaking in acetone, as this can strip away the remaining moisture from an already stressed nail bed.

We have to talk about "photosensitivity"—a fancy way of saying your skin has become a sponge for sunlight. Many lymphoma medications make your skin significantly more prone to burning, even on a cloudy day or through a window. This isn't just about avoiding a tan; it's about protecting skin that is currently less able to repair itself from UV damage. A broad-spectrum SPF 30 or higher should become as much a part of your daily routine as brushing your teeth. Combined with a wide-brimmed hat and lightweight long sleeves, this "sun-armor" ensures that you can still enjoy being outdoors without paying for it with a painful burn later. By treating your external self with the same strategic care you give your internal health, you aren't just managing side effects; you are honoring the vessel that is carrying you through this process, ensuring that as you heal within, your "external journey" is as comfortable as possible.

CHAPTER 21: MOUTH SORES AND TASTE CHANGES

One of the most intimate challenges of the lymphoma journey is when the very act of eating —something that should be a source of comfort and strength—becomes a source of frustration. This usually happens because the lining of the mouth and the taste buds are composed of fast-dividing cells, making them accidental targets for many systemic treatments. The result is often twofold: the development of painful mouth sores, known as mucositis, and a strange, persistent distortion of flavor frequently described as "metallic mouth." It can feel as though your palate has been hijacked, turning a favorite meal into something that tastes like tinfoil or cardboard.

To manage mouth sores, the goal is to create a "peace treaty" with your oral environment. When the lining of the mouth is thin or inflamed, every bite can feel like it's being rubbed with sandpaper. This is the time to embrace soft, "slippery" foods. Think of things that require very little chewing and can slide down easily, like Greek yogurt, well-blended smoothies, or mashed potatoes thinned with a bit of broth. You should also avoid the "irritant triad": acid, salt, and spice. Even a squeeze of lemon or a dash of black pepper that would normally be invisible can feel like a fire in a sensitized mouth. Instead, focus on "cooling" sensations—sucking on ice chips or frozen fruit popsicles can provide a temporary numbing effect that makes the next few bites of a meal much more tolerable.

The "metallic mouth" or taste changes require a bit more creativity, almost like a chemistry experiment in your own kitchen. If everything tastes like metal, the secret is often to use "plastic" or "bamboo" utensils. It sounds overly simple, but avoiding metal silverware can significantly reduce the metallic tang that your brain is perceiving. If foods taste too sweet or "cloying," adding a tiny bit of salt or a drop of lemon juice (provided you don't have active sores) can help balance the scales. Conversely, if everything tastes bitter, a small amount of honey or maple syrup can mask those harsh notes. Many people find that tart flavors—like a bit of pickled ginger or a lemon drop—can "reset" the palate before a meal, clearing out the lingering metallic taste so the actual flavor of the food has a chance to shine through.

Oral hygiene also plays a surprisingly large role in how things taste. A clean mouth simply functions better. However, you have to ditch the "alcohol-based" mouthwashes that sting and dry out the tissues. Instead, many oncologists recommend a simple, homemade "salt and soda" rinse—just a half-teaspoon of salt and a half-teaspoon of baking soda in a glass of warm water. Rinsing with this several times a day helps neutralize the acid in your mouth, keeps the sores clean, and can actually help clear away some of the "fuzziness" that contributes to taste changes. It's a gentle, effective way to maintain the "garden" of your mouth while it's under stress.

Reclaiming the joy of eating is about small victories. It's about finding that one "safe" food that still tastes like it should—maybe it's a cold piece of watermelon or a simple bowl of rice—and leaning into it without guilt. Your nutritional needs are high right now, but so is your need for a bit of pleasure. By managing the physical discomfort with gentle choices and "outsmarting" the taste distortions with clever flavor balancing, you aren't just getting through treatment; you are protecting your relationship with one of life's most fundamental joys.

CHAPTER 22: THE "WATCH AND WAIT" PARADOX

The term "Watch and Wait" is perhaps the most linguistically deceptive phrase in all of medicine. To an outsider, it sounds like a period of reprieve, a gentle grace period where one can simply put the diagnosis on a shelf and get back to living. But for the person actually inhabiting that space, it often feels more like a "Watch and Worry" paradox. You are essentially being asked to coexist with an uninvited guest—one you know is there, yet one your medical team is choosing not to evict just yet. It is the psychological equivalent of being told there is a small, slow-moving fire in the attic, but that the fire department recommends just checking on it every few months rather than spraying it with water.

This creates a unique mental friction. In almost every other aspect of life, we are taught that action equals progress. If a tooth aches, you fill the cavity; if a car engine knocks, you take it to the mechanic. Being told that "doing nothing" is the most aggressive and sophisticated way to protect your long-term health feels fundamentally counterintuitive. This dissonance often leads to what many in the community call "scanxiety"—that creeping sense of dread that begins weeks before a follow-up appointment, where every minor ache, every slightly itchy patch of skin, or every night you wake up a bit warm becomes a potential piece of evidence that the "peace treaty" has been broken.

To manage this burden, you have to shift your perspective on what "Active Surveillance" actually is. It is not a passive state of ignoring the disease; it is a highly disciplined form of medical observation. You are not "waiting for the other shoe to drop"; you are waiting for the optimal moment to intervene, ensuring that when you do use your medical ammunition, it is at its most effective. One of the most helpful ways to lower the temperature of this anxiety is to "compartmentalize" the lymphoma. You might decide that the lymphoma is only allowed to have your attention during the week of your blood work and scans. The rest of the time, it is relegated to the background, much like a background app on a phone that is running but not draining the battery of your daily life.

It also helps to acknowledge that your feelings are a completely rational response to an irrational situation. You aren't "being dramatic" or "failing at being positive." You are navigating a sophisticated form of long-term uncertainty. Many people find relief in the "Three-Day Rule": give yourself permission to be a "professional patient" for three days around your appointments—worry, ask the tough questions, and feel the weight of it—but then, once the data is in and the plan for the next six months is set, consciously step back into your "civilian" life.

Living well in the paradox also requires a shift in how we talk about "the enemy." When we use battle metaphors—fighting, winning, losing—we set up a binary where anything other than total eradication feels like defeat. In follicular lymphoma, a more helpful analogy is that of a "managed ecosystem." You are the steward of that ecosystem. Sometimes the weeds are present, but the garden is still beautiful and functional. By focusing on the "and"— I have follicular lymphoma *and* I am living a full, vibrant life—you strip the disease of its power to be the only story you tell about yourself. You aren't ignoring the fire in the attic; you've simply decided that as long as the floorboards aren't hot, you're still going to host the dinner party downstairs.

CHAPTER 23: SCANXIETY: NAVIGATING THE TWO-WEEK WAIT

"Scanxiety" is a term that isn't found in any medical textbook, but for anyone living with follicular lymphoma, it is a diagnosis as real as the one on their pathology report. It describes that specific, high-voltage tension that begins the moment a follow-up PET or CT scan is scheduled and doesn't discharge until the doctor finally says, "Everything looks stable." This "two-week wait"—spanning the days leading up to the scan and the agonizing silence while waiting for the results—can feel like a glitch in time, where the future is put on hold and your mind becomes a master of "worst-case scenario" architecture.

To navigate this period, you have to realize that scanxiety is essentially a survival mechanism gone into overdrive. Your brain is trying to protect you by preparing for every possible outcome, but in doing so, it often robs you of the present. One of the most effective ways to ground yourself is to practice what I call "radical scheduling." Instead of letting the anxiety bleed into every hour of your day, give it a dedicated time slot. Decide that from 4:00 to 4:30 PM, you are allowed to worry, Google your symptoms, and feel the full weight of the uncertainty. When the timer goes off, you consciously pivot back to the task at hand. It sounds overly simple, but by giving the fear a "room" to live in, you prevent it from taking over the entire house.

The day of the scan itself often brings a unique sensory stress—the cold room, the hum of the machine, the "warm flush" of the contrast dye. It can help to view these elements not as clinical intruders, but as parts of a ritual. You are gathering the data that allows you to remain the CEO of your own health. Many people find comfort in "anchoring" themselves during the scan with a specific mental task. Perhaps you mentally recite the lyrics to a favorite album or visualize a place where you feel completely safe. By occupying the "verbal" or "visual" centers of your brain, you leave less room for the panic response to take root while you're inside the machine.

Then comes the real test: the wait for the results. In this phase, your imagination is your greatest enemy. It is incredibly common to experience "phantom symptoms"—suddenly feeling an ache in a node that was fine yesterday or convincing yourself that you're sweating more at night. This is your mind projecting its fears onto your body. When this happens, acknowledge the thought without necessarily believing it. Remind yourself: "I am feeling anxious, and anxiety can create physical sensations. These sensations are not the same as data." Until you have the scan report in front of you, everything else is just a story your mind is telling to fill the silence.

It also helps to be very clear with your medical team about *how* you want to receive your results. Do you want a phone call as soon as they're in, or do you prefer to wait for an in-person appointment where you can look at the images together? Knowing exactly when and how the information will arrive can shorten the "wait time" and give you a sense of agency. If you use a patient portal where results are posted automatically, decide ahead of time if you actually want to look at them before talking to your doctor. Sometimes, reading a radiologist's technical notes without context can create more fear than clarity.

Navigating the two-week wait is about being incredibly kind to yourself. This is the time to lower your expectations for productivity and raise your commitment to self-care. Watch the movies that make you laugh, spend time with people who don't ask you how you're "feeling" every five minutes, and move your body in ways that feel good. You are more than a set of images on a screen, and regardless of what the "pixels" show, you have already developed the resilience to meet whatever comes next. The scan is just a map; you are the one driving the car.

CHAPTER 24: DIFFICULT CONVERSATIONS: TALKING TO FAMILY AND CHILDREN

One of the most daunting tasks after a diagnosis of follicular lymphoma isn't the treatment or the scans—it's the weight of the words you have to say to the people you love. There is a profound sense of responsibility that comes with sharing this news, particularly when you're explaining a condition that doesn't fit the "standard" cancer narrative. Because follicular lymphoma is often chronic and indolent, you aren't just breaking bad news; you are teaching your family how to live with a new, long-term reality. The goal of these conversations isn't to provide a medical lecture, but to offer a clear, calm, and honest framework that allows your loved ones to feel secure even in the face of uncertainty.

When talking to adult family members or partners, the biggest hurdle is often correcting the immediate assumption that you are in a life-or-death crisis. Most people hear the word "cancer" and think of a sprint—an immediate, aggressive battle. You have to gently shift them toward the marathon. A helpful way to frame this is by using the "chronic condition" analogy. You might say, "I have a type of lymphoma that the doctors describe as a slow-moving, chronic condition. It's more like having something like diabetes than a typical fast-moving cancer. It's something we're going to manage over many years, and right now, the plan is to monitor it closely rather than jump into heavy treatment." This phrasing provides the "what" and the "why" simultaneously, offering a sense of control that lowers the collective temperature of the room.

Talking to children, especially younger ones like an eight-year-old, requires a different kind of precision. Children are incredibly perceptive; they can feel the "static" in the air even if they don't understand the source. If you don't give them a story, they will often invent one that is far scarier than the truth. For a child, keep it concrete and focus on the "now." You might explain it by saying, "You know how our bodies have a tiny army inside that fights off colds? Well, a small part of my army is a little confused and is growing too many cells in my lymph nodes —those little bumps you can sometimes feel in your neck. The good news is that this is a very slow-moving 'glitch,' and the doctors are experts at watching it. I'm not 'sick' in the way you are when you have the flu, and I can still do all the things we love to do together." This validates their observations without overwhelming them with a future they can't yet grasp.

It is also important to address the "why aren't you doing anything?" question, which often comes from a place of love and anxiety. Well-meaning relatives might push for "second opinions" or "aggressive" alternatives because they want to see you "fighting."

For these moments, having a script helps you maintain your own boundaries. You can say, "I know it feels strange that we aren't starting treatment today, but the best medical strategy for this specific type of lymphoma is to save the strong medicines for when they are truly needed. Right now, my body is doing great on its own, and 'watching' is actually the most active thing we can do to protect my health long-term." This centers the conversation on strategy rather than passivity.

These conversations are less about the words you choose and more about the "emotional tone" you set. If you can speak with a grounded, approachable confidence, your family will take their cues from you. It's okay to say "I don't know" when a question hits a gray area—in fact, it's better to be honest about the uncertainty than to offer false certainty. By inviting your family into the "chronic" mindset, you transform them from worried bystanders into a supportive team. You are showing them that while the diagnosis is a part of your life, it isn't the whole story, and that together, you have plenty of time to navigate the chapters ahead.

CHAPTER 25: INTIMACY AND SEXUALITY DURING TREATMENT

Of all the topics we've discussed in this journey through follicular lymphoma, intimacy is perhaps the one most often left behind in the doctor's office. There is a tendency to focus so intently on blood counts, scans, and treatment cycles that we forget about the quietest part of the diagnosis: the way it changes how we relate to the person we love. Intimacy is a delicate ecosystem of physical desire and emotional safety, and a chronic diagnosis—along with the treatments that follow—can feel like a series of tremors moving through that ground. It isn't just about the physical act of sex; it's about the shift from being "partners" to being "patient and caregiver," and the complicated work of finding your way back to each other.

The most immediate hurdle is often physical. We've talked about the "Spoon Theory" in terms of daily chores, but it applies just as strictly to your romantic life. Fatigue is a profound "desire-killer." When you are using every ounce of energy just to navigate the day, the idea of physical intimacy can feel like another exhausting task on an already too-long list. This is compounded by the "collateral damage" of treatment: the skin sensitivity we discussed in the external journey, the "metallic mouth" that can make kissing feel strange, or the hormonal shifts triggered by steroids and chemotherapy that can dampen libido or cause physical discomfort. It's important to recognize that these aren't "failures" of your relationship; they are biological side effects. Your body is currently prioritizing survival and repair, and sometimes that means the systems responsible for desire are temporarily placed on "low-power mode."

Beyond the biological, there is the significant hurdle of body image. It is difficult to feel sensual when you don't quite recognize the person in the mirror. Whether it's the thinning hair, the "Rituximab rash," or the "moon face" caused by steroids, these changes can make you feel exposed and vulnerable in a way that isn't particularly romantic. You might find yourself pulling away from your partner's touch, not because you don't love them, but because you don't feel "loveable" in that moment. On the other side of the equation, your partner might be pulling away out of fear—the fear of causing you pain, the fear of "doing something wrong," or even a misplaced worry about the safety of physical contact during treatment. These silent assumptions can create a vast, chilly distance in the bedroom if they aren't brought out into the light.

The secret to navigating this "new normal" is the art of redefinition. We have to broaden our definition of intimacy to include everything from a long, quiet hug to simply sitting together in the garden. If the "sexual" isn't possible today because of fatigue or discomfort, the "sensual" is still very much available. This might mean a gentle foot rub for those aching, neuropathic feet, or a scalp massage to soothe the sensitivity of thinning hair. By shifting the goal from "performance" to "connection," you take the pressure off yourself and your partner. You are essentially telling the lymphoma that while it can influence your energy, it does not get to dictate your closeness.

Communication, as cliché as it sounds, is the only bridge across this gap. You have to be willing to have the "uncomfortable" conversations. This means being honest when you're too tired, but also being clear that your lack of desire isn't a lack of love. A helpful way to frame this is to say, "I really want to be close to you tonight, but my body feels very drained. Can we just hold each other while we watch a movie instead?" For the partner, it means asking, "I want to be close to you, but I'm worried about hurting you—tell me what feels good today." These small, vulnerable check-ins prevent resentment from building and ensure that the "caregiver" role doesn't completely swallow the "lover" role.

Intimacy during treatment is a form of resilience. It is an assertion that you are still a whole person with needs, desires, and a capacity for connection that exists independently of your diagnosis. It requires patience, a good sense of humor, and a willingness to explore new ways of being together. As you move through the chapters of recovery and remission, your physical energy will return, and the fog of treatment will lift. In the meantime, protecting that core connection with your partner is one of the most powerful ways to remind yourself of who you are beyond the patient ID bracelet.

CHAPTER 26: THE ORGANIZED PATIENT: MANAGING RECORDS AND RESULTS

One of the most empowering shifts you can make on this journey is moving from being a passive recipient of medical news to becoming the chief archivist of your own health. When you are dealing with a chronic condition like follicular lymphoma, the sheer volume of data—biopsy reports, blood counts, imaging discs, and treatment summaries—can quickly become an avalanche. Relying on a hospital's digital portal is a good start, but those portals are often fragmented, and they don't always speak to each other. Building your own "Lymphoma Binder" is about more than just staying organized; it is about creating a central "source of truth" that allows you to walk into any consultation with the confidence of someone who has the full map spread out in front of them.

Think of your binder as the "black box" flight recorder for your treatment. The foundation of this archive should be your pathology and biopsy results. These are the "birth certificates" of your diagnosis, containing the specific markers like CD20 and Ki-67 that we discussed earlier. Having hard copies of these is essential because if you ever seek a second opinion or travel to a new specialist, these are the first things they will need to see to understand the "personality" of your lymphoma. Behind these, you'll want to keep your imaging reports—the written summaries of your CT or PET scans. While the actual discs are important, the written reports provide the chronological narrative of how your lymph nodes have changed over time, allowing you to spot trends that might not be obvious in a single snapshot.

The most dynamic part of your binder, however, will be your blood work. In follicular lymphoma, we track specific numbers like your Absolute Neutrophil Count (ANC), hemoglobin, and platelets with the vigilance of a hawk. Rather than just filing these away, I highly recommend creating a simple "flow sheet" or a tracking graph. When you see your counts plotted on a line over several months, you can visualize the "dips" during treatment and the "climbs" during recovery. It transforms a list of confusing numbers into a clear picture of your body's resilience. It also helps you identify your own "normal"—you might learn that your body naturally runs a bit lower on certain counts than the laboratory's generic average, which can save you a lot of unnecessary worry.

Beyond the clinical data, your binder should also function as a "symptom and side effect" journal. This doesn't need to be an exhaustive diary, but a quick daily or weekly log of how you're feeling. Did the "queasies" peak on day three after the infusion? Did the neuropathy in your feet flare up when it rained? By recording these patterns, you can provide your oncology team with high-quality "intelligence." Instead of saying "I've been feeling tired," you can say, "I've noticed my fatigue hits its wall around 2:00 PM every Tuesday, but I feel much better by Friday." This level of detail allows your doctor to fine-tune your supportive care—adjusting the timing of anti-nausea meds or steroids to better fit your body's specific rhythm.

Dedicate a section of your binder to the "Questions for Next Time." We've all had that experience where we have a dozen burning questions at home, only for our minds to go blank the moment the doctor walks into the exam room. Keeping a running list ensures that no concern is too small to be addressed. Your binder is a physical manifestation of your agency; it says that while you cannot control the genetics of your B-cells, you are in total control of the strategy used to manage them. It turns a chaotic medical experience into a manageable project, providing a sense of order that is often the best antidote to the uncertainty of a chronic diagnosis.

CHAPTER 27: CAREER AND CANCER: TO WORK OR NOT TO WORK?

Deciding whether to continue working after a follicular lymphoma diagnosis is rarely a simple "yes" or "no" question; it is a complex, evolving negotiation between your physical needs, your financial reality, and your sense of identity. For many, work is more than just a paycheck—it is a tether to "normalcy," a place where you are a colleague or a leader rather than a patient. However, follicular lymphoma is a marathon, and the way you approach your career has to shift from a sprint to a long-term endurance strategy. You don't have to make all these decisions on day one, but understanding the safety net beneath you can turn a panic-driven choice into a deliberate, empowered plan.

In the early stages, particularly during "Watch and Wait," many people find that staying at work is actually their best medicine. It provides structure and keeps the mind occupied. But if and when treatment begins, the landscape changes. This is where you should look into the legal protections available to you, specifically the Americans with Disabilities Act (ADA) and the Family and Medical Leave Act (FMLA). Under the ADA, a cancer diagnosis is generally considered a disability, which grants you the right to "reasonable accommodations." This isn't about asking for special treatment; it's about leveling the playing field. It might mean a more ergonomic chair to help with neuropathic pain, the ability to work from home on days when your "spoon budget" is low, or a flexible schedule that allows for those mid-morning infusions. These adjustments are designed to keep you productive without draining your battery to zero.

If the fatigue or the treatment schedule becomes too heavy to manage even with accommodations, FMLA is your most powerful tool. It allows you to take up to twelve weeks of unpaid, job-protected leave per year. The beauty of FMLA is that it doesn't have to be taken all at once. You can use it "intermittently"—taking a day off here for a scan or a few days there for a treatment cycle—while knowing your position and your health insurance remain secure. It's a vital pressure valve that prevents you from having to choose between your health and your livelihood. Before you have "the talk" with Human Resources, take some time to review your employee handbook. Look specifically at your short-term and long-term disability policies, as these are the financial bridges that can help if you need to step away for an extended period.

The "when" and "how" of disclosing your diagnosis to your employer is a deeply personal choice. You are under no legal obligation to share every detail of your pathology report. In many cases, a simple note from your doctor stating that you have a "chronic medical condition" requiring certain accommodations is enough to trigger your legal protections. When you do speak with your manager, try to frame the conversation around solutions rather than limitations. Instead of saying, "I can't do this anymore," try, "I want to remain a productive part of this team, and to do that, I'll need a bit of flexibility with my start times on treatment weeks." This approach preserves your professional standing while clearly communicating your needs.

Your career is a part of your life, but it isn't your whole life. There may be seasons where your work takes a back seat so that your recovery can take the wheel, and that is not a failure—it's a tactical retreat. By using the legal and organizational tools at your disposal, you can manage your professional identity in a way that respects your body's new rhythm. Whether you choose to work through treatment or take a much-needed hiatus, the goal is to ensure that your career remains a choice you make, rather than a burden you're forced to carry.

CHAPTER 28: THE LYMPHOMA TRAVELER'S GUIDE

For many people living with follicular lymphoma, the diagnosis can feel like an invisible tether, grounding you to your home clinic and your local pharmacy. But the truth is that the "indolent" nature of this disease often allows for a high quality of life that includes seeing the world. Whether you're in a quiet period of "Watch and Wait" or you've successfully navigated treatment, traveling is not only possible—it can be a vital part of reclaiming your sense of self. However, traveling with a "confused" immune system requires moving away from the "winging it" mentality of your younger years and toward a more strategic, well-provisioned approach. Think of yourself as a high-value envoy: you can go anywhere, but you need the right clearances and a very specific survival kit.

The first stop on your itinerary should always be your oncologist's office, ideally six to eight weeks before you depart. This is about more than just a "green light" for the trip; it's about the complex world of vaccinations. For a lymphoma traveler, vaccines are divided into two categories: "safe" and "no-go." Most routine travel vaccines, like those for Hepatitis A or Typhoid, are inactivated (killed) and are generally safe, though they may be slightly less effective if your immune system is currently suppressed. However, "live" vaccines—such as those for Yellow Fever, Measles, or the nasal spray version of the flu vaccine—contain a weakened but living virus. If you are immunocompromised, these can be dangerous. If your destination requires a live vaccine for entry, your doctor may need to provide a formal "waiver" letter, or you may need to reconsider that specific location in favor of one with fewer biological hurdles.

When it comes to the logistics of the journey, your carry-on bag is your fortress. Never, under any circumstances, pack your essential medications in checked luggage. Between the risk of lost bags and the extreme temperature fluctuations in a plane's cargo hold, it's a gamble you don't need to take. Keep all medications in their original, labeled pharmacy bottles. This isn't just for organization; it's for customs and security. If you are traveling internationally, carry a "letter of medical necessity" from your doctor that lists every medication, including any injectable supplies like syringes or cooling packs for temperature-sensitive drugs. This letter is your "get out of jail free" card at security checkpoints, ensuring that your "liquid" medications are treated as the essential tools they are.

Flying itself presents a few unique challenges for the lymphoma patient. The recycled air in a cabin is a playground for germs, and when your neutrophil counts are low, a minor cold can become a major event. This is the time to be the person in the N95 mask. It's also the time to stay mobile. Lymphoma and its treatments can slightly increase the risk of blood clots during long periods of immobility. Secure an aisle seat, stay hydrated with bottled water, and make it a habit to get up and walk for five minutes every hour. If your "spoon budget" is low, don't be afraid to request airport assistance or a wheelchair; saving your energy for the destination is a much better strategy than exhausting yourself in the security line.

Once you arrive, your "lymphoma-friendly kitchen" rules travel with you. Be the "safe water" advocate: stick to bottled water for drinking and even for brushing your teeth in areas where water quality is questionable. Avoid the siren call of the open buffet or the street food stall where items have been sitting out. If you're traveling to a sunny or tropical locale, remember that many lymphoma treatments make your skin a "sun sponge." Pack a wide-brimmed hat, long sleeves, and a high-SPF sunscreen as if they are part of your prescription. By being a vigilant, well-prepared traveler, you turn the "tether" of the diagnosis into a long, flexible lead—allowing you to explore the world while knowing your "inner castle" remains securely protected.

CHAPTER 29: FINANCIAL TOXICITY: NAVIGATING INSURANCE AND ASSISTANCE

One of the most jarring realizations after a follicular lymphoma diagnosis is that the disease doesn't just inhabit your body; it also enters your bank account. In the medical world, we have a term for this: "financial toxicity." It's a clinical-sounding name for a very raw and stressful reality —the way the cost of chronic care can erode a family's stability just as surely as the disease itself. When you're dealing with high-cost biologics like rituximab or the newer "frontier" treatments, even with decent insurance, the out-of-pocket costs can be staggering. Navigating this isn't just about bookkeeping; it's about learning to advocate for your financial health with the same tenacity you use for your physical recovery.

The first thing to understand is that the "sticker price" of cancer care is rarely what you are actually meant to pay. The healthcare system is a labyrinth of negotiated rates, and your first line of defense is a deep understanding of your insurance policy's "maximum out-of-pocket" (MOOP) limit. This is the ceiling on what you have to pay in a calendar year for covered, in-network services. Once you hit that number, the insurance company picks up 100% of the cost. In follicular lymphoma, where treatment can be expensive, many patients hit this limit quite early in the year. Knowing this number allows you to plan your "financial spoons," understanding that while the beginning of the year is expensive, the latter half will likely be covered.

However, even reaching that ceiling can be a struggle, and this is where "copay cards" and "foundation grants" come into play. Most pharmaceutical companies that manufacture specialty lymphoma drugs offer patient assistance programs. If you are on a branded medication, the manufacturer often provides a copay card that can bring your cost down to as little as five or ten dollars. These cards aren't based on your income; they are designed to bypass the high cost of the drug so that you can access the treatment you need. It's always worth a five-minute search on the drug manufacturer's website or a quick call to their patient support line. It's essentially a "coupon" for life-saving medicine, and there is no shame in using every tool available to you.

For the costs that insurance and copay cards don't cover—like office visits, scans, or travel expenses—there are non-profit foundations. Organizations like the Leukemia & Lymphoma Society (LLS) or the Patient Access Network (PAN) Foundation offer grants specifically for follicular lymphoma patients. These are often based on financial need, but the thresholds are usually more generous than you might expect. These funds can be a lifesaver for those "invisible" costs of cancer, like transportation to the clinic or the high price of supportive medications. The key here is timing; these funds are often first-come, first-served and can open and close throughout the year. Setting an alert or having a family member check these sites once a month can make the difference between a bill you can handle and one that feels impossible.

We have to talk about the actual medical bills. It's important to remember that a bill is just an opening statement, not a final verdict. Errors in medical billing are incredibly common—it might be a double-charge for a lab test or a "denied" claim that simply needs a different coding from your doctor's office. Never pay a large, confusing bill without first requesting an "itemized statement" and comparing it to your insurance "Explanation of Benefits" (EOB). If the numbers don't match, don't panic. Call the hospital's billing department and ask to speak with a financial counselor. Most hospitals have "charity care" policies or payment plans that can significantly reduce the burden. They would much rather work out a manageable monthly payment with you than have the bill go to collections.

Managing financial toxicity is about recognizing that you are a consumer in a very complex marketplace. It's okay to ask, "How much will this scan cost?" or "Is there a generic version of this supportive medication?" Being a "financially organized" patient—keeping your EOBs in that

Lymphoma Binder we discussed and staying on top of assistance deadlines—removes the element of surprise. By tackling the costs with a strategy, you ensure that your focus remains where it belongs: on your healing, your family, and your future.

CHAPTER 30: THE CAREGIVER'S COMPASS

In the landscape of follicular lymphoma, if the patient is the one navigating the terrain, the caregiver is the compass—the steady, orienting force that keeps the journey on track. But being a compass is exhausting work. It requires a constant, quiet expenditure of emotional and physical energy that often goes unnoticed until the needle begins to flicker. We talk a lot about "patient burnout," but caregiver burnout is just as real and, in some ways, more insidious. Because your focus is so intently fixed on your loved one, you may not notice your own "battery" draining until you are running on empty, feeling a sense of resentment, exhaustion, or a heavy, foggy detachment that you don't quite recognize.

The first step in preventing this burnout is to dismantle the myth of the "Selfless Caregiver." There is a pervasive idea that to truly love someone with a chronic illness, you must put your own needs entirely on the back burner. In reality, this is a recipe for disaster. Think of the safety briefing on an airplane: you must put on your own oxygen mask before helping others. If you are gasping for air, you are of no use to the person sitting next to you. Taking time for a walk, a quiet cup of coffee, or a night out with friends isn't "selfish"; it is a vital act of maintenance that ensures you remain a capable, resilient partner in this marathon.

To navigate the path without losing yourself, you have to become an expert at the art of delegation. Most caregivers fall into the trap of trying to do everything—the cooking, the cleaning, the insurance calls, and the emotional heavy lifting—because they feel they are the only ones who "know the routine." But you have to remember that people around you often want to help but don't know how. When a friend asks, "What can I do?", don't give the reflexive "Nothing, we're fine." Instead, give them a specific, "low-stakes" task from your list. Ask them to pick up the dry cleaning, walk the dog for thirty minutes, or drop off a rotisserie chicken. By offloading these small tasks, you preserve your "emotional spoons" for the things that only you can do: being the source of comfort and the keeper of the shared history.

We also have to address the "Emotional Echo." When your partner is having a hard day—perhaps they are dealing with "the queasies" or a flare-up of scanxiety—it is natural for you to feel those emotions too. But you have to learn to distinguish between empathy and absorption. You can be a supportive witness to their pain without having to inhabit it yourself. This requires building a "parallel support system." You need a space where you are not "The Caregiver," but simply yourself. Whether it's a support group specifically for partners, a therapist, or a trusted friend who can talk about anything *except* lymphoma, having a place to vent your own frustrations, fears, and even your "caregiver guilt" is essential for keeping your own internal compass calibrated.

Give yourself the grace of the "Good Enough" rule. There will be days when the house is a mess, the laundry is piled high, and you ordered takeout for the third night in a row. In the grand scheme of a follicular lymphoma journey, these things do not matter. What matters is the connection between you and your loved one. If you are both safe, fed, and together, you have succeeded. By lowering the bar for the "logistics" of life, you leave more room for the moments of joy, humor, and quiet closeness that are the real fuel for the road ahead. You are walking a difficult path, but you aren't walking it alone, and your well-being is every bit as important as the person you are caring for.

ABOUT THE AUTHOR

Dr. Bhratri Bhushan

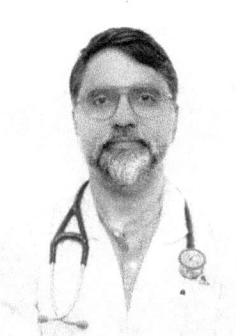

Dr. Bhratri Bhushan is a Consultant Medical Oncologist and Hematologist dedicated to bridging the gap between complex medical science and patient understanding. Combining his clinical expertise with a passion for education, he has authored multiple books on oncology and internal medicine designed to empower readers with knowledge. His research is widely recognized and has been published in renowned international medical journals. You can find his full collection of books and guides at www.amazon.com/author/bhratribhushan

www.ingramcontent.com/pod-product-compliance
Lightning Source LLC
Chambersburg PA
CBHW052323220526
45472CB00001B/250